W9-CJM-769

Back
Works

by

Timothy J. Gray, D.O.

BookPartners, Inc.
Seattle, Washington

Advil is a registered trademark of WhiteHall Laboratories, New York, New York.
Nuprin is a registered trademark of Bristol Laboratories, Evansville, Indiana.
Thera-Band is a registered trademark of The Hygenic Corporation, Akron, Ohio.
Cybex is a registered trademark of Cybex Corporation, Ronkonkoma, New York.
Nautilus is a registered trademark of Nautilus Corporation, Independence, Virginia.
Kevlar is a registered trademark of E.I. DuPont Corporation, Wilmington, Delaware.
Medx is a registered trademark of Medx Corporation, Ocala, Florida.
Cytotec is a registered trademark of Searle Corporation, Chicago, Illinois.
Porsche is a registered trademark of Dr. Ing H.C.F. Porsche, Stuttgart, Germany.
Medipren is a registered trademark of McNeil Corporation, Fort Washington, PA.
Ace Hardware is a registered trademark of Ace Hardware Corporation, Oak Brook, IL.
NordicTrack is a registered trademark of NordicTrack, Chaska, Minnesota.
Goretex is a registered trademark of Gore and Associates, Newark, Delaware.
Didronel is a registered trademark of MGI Pharmaceuticals, Minneapolis, Minnesota.
Kincom is a registered trademark of Chatteck Corporation, Chattanooga, Tennessee.
Lido is a registered trademark of Loredan, Inc., Davis, California.

DECATUR PUBLIC LIBRARY

SEP 15 1993

DECATUR, ILLINOIS

WITHDRAWN

Copyright 1993 by Dr. Timothy Gray.
All Rights reserved
Library of Congress Catalog 92-063045
ISBN 0-9622269-1-2

This book may not be reproduced in whole or in part, by mimeograph or any other
means, without permission. For information address:

BookPartners, Inc.

P.O. Box 19732
Seattle, Washington 98109

Dedication

*This book is dedicated to my wife Kathy
and to our children T.J., Tom and Laura.*

Acknowledgments

I would like to personally thank Thorn and Ursula Bacon for their editing and organizational skills throughout the production of this book.

In addition a special thanks to Gracie Campbell who illustrated the text and brought the concepts to life.

To Jenine Vrtiska thank you for coordinating activities at Spinecare Of The Pacific.

A thank you to the giants in spine medicine, Arthur White, Arthur Jones, W. H. Kirkaldy-Willis, Tom Mayer, Robert Gatchel, Jeff and Joel Saal, Vijay Goel and James Weinstein whose research served as a stimulus for this book.

Table Of Contents

1. Exercise Is The Key To A Healthy Back 1
   Strengthening, stretching and aerobic activity
   keep supporting muscles fit.

2. Spine Aging Occurs With Inactivity 7
   Three sets of exercises prevent back trouble;
   discover your fitness with the back flexibility test.

3. Well-defined Backs Are Built, Not Born 29
   Exercise ten minutes a day
   to offset office fatigue and tone muscles.

4. Four Out Of Five Of Us Will Experience Back Trouble.......42
   Physical neglect is the prime reason
   people see a physician or chiropractor.

5. How Do You Judge The Seriousness Of A Back Attack? 62
   Read about the rule of thumb that tells you
   when you should try a home remedy to relieve pain.

6. The "Bad" Reputation Of Herniated Or Ruptured Discs 79
   It's not true that ruptures always
   prevent people from sports or heavy work.

7. Osteoporosis And Back Pain—Fragile And Frail Bones......93
   A preventable disease that makes women susceptible
   to hip and vertebrae fractures.

8. First Aid For Flare Ups—Keeping Active 105
    You can relieve pain from back aches,
    then use stretching to stop muscle spasms.

9. Armor-Plating The Spine 123
    Toughened muscles will shield your
    back from routine injuries.

10. Building Endurance And Performance 131
    Back exercise machines are designed to stress
    muscle groups that strengthen the spine.

11. Stretching Stops Pain 140
    The household cat knows how to flex rest-softened
    muscles, making them relax.

12. Aerobics 150
    Creating strength, flexibility and endurance through
    exercises that increase heart rate.

13. Age Vigorously Or Age Rapidly... 157
    Older people are proving fitness can improve
    longevity and physical agility.

14. Antigravity Exercises For The Elderly............................... 168
    Muscle strength can be tripled
    in people thought to be too old to stay active.

15. Questions I Am Frequently Asked By
    Back Pain Patients.. 175
    Don't be surprised at some of the answers;
    they prove the back can be trained to recover from inury.

< 1 >

Exercise Is The Key To A Healthy Back

Strengthening, stretching and aerobic activity
keep supporting muscles fit.

If you're worried about your back, if you've had uncertain twinges, stiffness, occasional streaks of pain or feelings of weakness, you'll be glad you bought this book. It will help you immediately if you're in pain. If you are among the 20 percent of Americans who have strong and healthy backs, congratulations. The book will show you how to prevent your back from "acting up".

There is no secret about the message in this book. It is based on the exercise treatments devised by the author for hundreds of his patients. These "prescription exercises" work. They can be performed in the home. They can transform a depressed back patient into a smiling, functioning person in a few months. In a matter of days, progress can be measured as weak, tense muscles are rejuvenated and the cloud of gloom and pain that hovers over the back-injured person disappears.

A symbol of strength, character and confidence, the back not only supports the physical apparatus of the human body, it reflects the mental and spiritual states of a person's health. That's why back pain is so debilitating. It's an attack from behind, from an area you can't defend. When your back hurts, you're vulnerable. You feel as if you've been let down, victimized. And you have. We're all exposed to emotional and mechanical stresses every day of our lives. If our backs aren't strong and supportive, we're in trouble.

Some of these stresses are unavoidable. Humans aren't meant to stand upright or sit in chairs, so we're fighting gravity all of the time. Just moving through the day—bending, lifting, carrying—can present unexpected hazards. If your back is in good condition, movements may not faze you. If it is not, you can be surprised by a simple injury that can lay you low, cause intolerable pain and convince you that maybe you "had it coming". Unfortunately, many physicians recommend lengthy bed rest and aspirin for a back injury. Not only, in the majority of cases, is the advice wrong, but it actually worsens the condition, prolonging the pain and reducing the strength, health and flexibility of the affected muscles. When the pain subsides and normal activities are resumed, the weakened back is more susceptible than ever to new injury.

Back problems cost the United States 60 billion dollars each year, and back pain is reported to be second only to sore throats as the most common ailment in the U.S. Although millions of people suffer from back pain, it is not the baffling malady it is represented to be.

Without question, more than 80 percent of all cases of back pain are caused by weak or tense muscles and not by an organic ailment, infection, or disease. This is incontrovertibly true.

Because weak, tense, unused muscles are responsible for the majority of all cases of back pain, we know they can be rehabilitated through a simple program of exercise. Almost invariably, pain is the result of the failure to use muscles properly and regularly.

Today it's not popular for physicians to make bold statements about restoring the health of a person in pain or promise the lack of pain by following a structured program. But, the fact is, I know that the prescription exercises I give in this book work because hundreds of my patients—in pain and agony as a result of injury to their out-of-condition-backs— have restored themselves to pain-free activities by following the simple exercise advice I give here. I call the process *Back Works* because that's what happens to more than 80 out of 100 people who perform the exercises and follow the advice we give in this book. The back starts working again the way it's supposed to. The exercises are designed to strengthen and improve the flexibility of key postural muscles in the body.

The axiom you should write down if you wish to avoid or minimize back trouble no matter what your age is : *Active people have less back pain.*

Vital to keeping your back healthy are these components: Good posture and alignment, weight control, adequate rest and stress management. You can accomplish these objectives by adopting an attitude of success and following the program I've developed. It involves:

1. Strengthening
2. Stretching
3. Aerobic activity

It seems to make sense, doesn't it, that there should be more emphasis on strengthening the torso—the mid-section and back—than the extremities? This was illustrated in a recent study of fire fighters—an occupation especially prone to back injuries—that showed that those who did back strength training have fewer back problems or injuries than those who don't.

A lack of flexibility can cause back problems also. For example, the hamstring muscles in the back of the thigh become inelastic when they get tight. An unexpected twist or turn pulls on the muscles above the hamstrings—in the lower back—so it's critical to keep them supple. Stretches and exercise maintain both in good condition.

Before we get into the SAFE Home Back Fitness Test and its components of strength, aerobics, flexibility and endurance in Chapter 2 of the book, it is worthwhile to understand why it is important to learn how to re-educate your body to help you move more efficiently and recover from and prevent injury to your back. Also we will look at a few simple do's and don'ts, and some hints for back health, which if heeded can make a remarkable difference in the condition of your back and in your mental view of the spine.

I cannot overemphasize the importance of aerobic activity. It strengthens the back and stomach, increases circulation and oxygen nourishment to the vertebral disks and promotes cardiovascular health. Aerobic activity also reduces stress, a major problem among back pain sufferers.

So strengthening, stretching and aerobic activity are the major keys to a strong healthy back. The exercises I recommend in this book combine these three requirements effectively. But, if you are like a lot of people you may hate to exercise. And, let's face it, strictly therapeutic exercises can be a crashing bore. Walk, swim, bicycle, play tennis regularly--just as long as you get the blood flowing. If you do these things faithfully, chances are you won't have to spend later years in pain. But even active people have to spend time in sedentary jobs with the result that in "unnatural" work situations stresses and strains are placed on the body that distort the back. As a result, you have to correct the harm. Walking and other brisk exercise are helpful, but may not completely restore the loss of muscle tone caused by tension, strain and fatigue.

Ideally, when you understand the simple procedures for keeping your back in action you should arrive at a point when you are always sensitive to your back's state of health and will do the things necessary to maintain it in good condition. This may be a combination of prescription exercises we give here and other enjoyable activities such as walking, swimming and tennis.

Posture is important to your back's health. Basically a good standing posture requires level, widened shoulders, a level slightly tucked pelvis, a lengthened—but not stiff—spine, relaxed knees and a tension-free lifted head. To put your head right, imagine a balloon with the string attached to the center of your skull pulling it up. You should be able to feel your shoulders drop and the sensation of your head floating. This takes a little practice, but it's worthwhile because correct posture will create better blood flow, sharpen your mind and improve your sense of well-being. Strengthening and stretching the back and hip muscles, and strengthening the stomach muscles will help hold your posture in place.

It is absolutely true that stress tightens and bunches muscles. We've discovered that people cannot always control the pressures in their lives, but can offset them with exercises and meditation. We discuss the physiological reason that exercise can release tension later in the book. Of course, getting adequate sleep seems obvious, but has generally been overlooked as a contributor to back health. Anytime you're awake, your muscles—whether you are moving or not--are contracting. You need rest in between. And how you sleep can be important to the relaxation of these muscles. Posture in bed depends on the sleep position that makes you most comfortable as long as the spine is supported.

Again, it may seem obvious, but staying within ten percent of your optimum weight is key to remaining back-pain free. Even more important is reduction of fat in the abdominal area. A big gut places pressure on the lower back and strains abdominal muscles past the point of efficiency. Spot reduction won't work; cutting down on fat intake and engaging in aerobic exercise will.

Despite attention to exercise and weight control, back injuries do happen. All injuries do not require a doctor's treatment. What do you do if your back goes out? These are the steps I recommend:

1. First assess the severity of the injury. If there is weakness or tingling in the legs, pain so severe that you can't sleep, a loss of bladder or bowel control, or if two days of self-treatment bring no relief, see a doctor.

2. For strain causing localized pain, lie down in a comfortable position on your side or back with your knees slightly bent. Place an ice pack against the painful area. The rule is ice for the first 48 hours to reduce swelling, then heat to relax the muscles. Don't plan on more than a couple of days of bed rest. That's enough.

Use aspirin or ibuprofen to reduce inflammation, at least two tablets every four hours—a somewhat higher dosage than usual. If you do see a doctor, don't go with the expectation that you'll be guaranteed a precise diagnosis of your pain. The sophisticated tools available now—ranging from X-rays to CAT scans to MRI—magnetic resonance imaging—can reveal a lot of things. When a disk, for example, puts pressure on nerve roots, this often causes a reaction known as sciatica, shooting pains down the leg. MRIs can show if there is a ruptured disk, a curvature of the backbone or a growth on the spine. But pain often exists without any visible cause. In some cases it persists after surgery has supposedly corrected the problem—the reason so many doctors recommend surgery as a last resort.

Avoidance of back problems, obviously, is the answer. Remember, you can put yourself into the 80 percent "good back health" category by following the prescription exercises in this book.

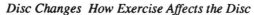

Disc Changes How Exercise Affects the Disc

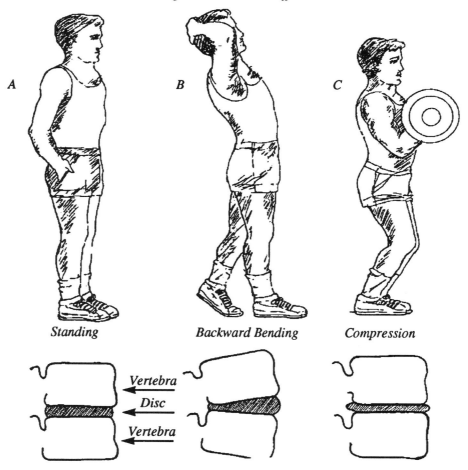

Side View of the Disc and Vertebrae

< 2 >

Spine Aging Occurs With Inactivity

*Three sets of exercises prevent back trouble;
discover your fitness with the back flexibility test.*

When I asked my back patients for their advice about where I should start in this book, overwhelmingly, they said, "Explain to your readers about the old-fashioned ideas in the medical system that result in the wrong treatment for people with back aches."

Tell them, they said, that prolonged rest is the worst thing they can do for a hurting back. Make them understand that failure to exercise is like giving your muscles a holiday or permission to go to sleep and to wither and withdraw their support from the spine. Without their support, the spine is like a flagpole that bends and creaks in the wind. Without strong, resilient muscles to hold and manage the spine, this column of sensitive bone loses body, character and flexibility.

Thousands of men and women in America are "spine-old" long before their time. Their backs, literally, age faster than other parts of their bodies as a result of neglect. Inevitably, other parts of the body begin to deteriorate when the back goes. It doesn't accomplish anything to blame medicine and doctors for being slow, and often resistant, to adopt new methods of caring for the back. It is a fact that many physicians still doggedly prescribe prolonged bed rest as the traditional response to a back injury, and it is also true that most of the books written about back care perpetuate the mistake of lengthy care to the detriment of people who have temporary back pain.

The message I want readers to understand is that there is only one major, accurate response to back pain and that is exercise. I have developed prescription exercises that restore the back to health. Performed, as they should be, before the back becomes troublesome, they prevent pain and lost time at work and play.

Pain has a devastating effect. It results in people doing what they often do in crisis—regressing to a more primitive method of dealing with life— pulling back and isolating themselves. Often they feel that the pain is their fault. Many of these people have been shuffled through the medical system and by the time they see a psychiatrist, still plagued with a back problem, they've been labeled as a difficult case or as a hypochondriac. Strangely, often these people have bypassed authentic programs of back strengthening that could have alleviated their pain.

When I see a patient who's been through the mill and has settled into a perpetual state of chronic misery, my first job is to convince him that he is not to blame for his situation but that there may be some patterns of mental and physical behavior perpetuating it. I devise a clear-cut plan, goals and objectives the patient can grasp. I help him to understand that, barring serious injury, disease or infection in his back, he can recover with effort and an exercise program that reduces his pain in a measurable way on a day to day basis. I tell my patients to forget miracles. Watch out for anyone, I advise, who promises a cure then signs you up for three sessions a week and doesn't give you any exercise. And be wary of a doctor who wants to operate immediately.

Never resort to drastic measures if there are other procedures to cure an injured back is my motto. I know exercise works, and I've selected the exercises that work best all of the time for this book. They start in Chapter 3. Just remember, back pain is just as preventative as tooth decay.

The exercises I describe in this book are divided into three categories:
1. Exercises for ten minutes a day to offset office fatigue.
2. Prescription exercises to armor-plate the back.
3. Specific exercises to restore particular back muscles.

Each of these sets is designed to perform a specific function. However, the ten minute exercises are designed only to counteract the effects of the sedentary office environment. They won't materially improve sports performance at the level of participation suggested nor will they always stop a nagging back ache. They are quite valuable, but the extent of their value will depend on the condition of your back when you start them. If you are in good shape, keeping active through healthy exercises such as walking, swimming, tennis, then these will be an added benefit to the fitness of your back.

If however, your back is out of shape, if you are an inactive person, are slow to exercise, or hate it, then they will start you on the road to an improved back. They should be initiated in conjunction with the SAFE Back Test in this chapter. If your total score is below 80, the ten minute exercises you'll find in Chapter 3 are not enough for you. You need to embark on the program of prescription exercises to armor-plate your back. Don't let this discourage you. Most of my patients score below 30 when they come to me, but their improvement is dramatic. You can determine the exact condition of your back and how much you have to do to get it in shape by taking the SAFE Test.

Most back pain is due to an unstable low back. The small muscles between the vertebrae become weak and allow the vertebrae to move beyond their normal limits and push against the nerves in the back. By strengthening these small muscles, the abnormal movement is prevented and the pain decreases. The SAFE back test is designed to show you how your back functions and points out your areas of strength and weakness. The initials

SAFE stand for strength, aerobics, flexibility and (muscular) endurance. The test measures the capability of your trunk muscles in the four functions described. As a result of taking the test, you will be able to keep a score card of your back health. Repeat the test monthly and watch your progress as you get your back working the way it should.

Who should take the test? Anyone age 14 or over can benefit from the test. Even 90-year-olds can increase their strength 300 percent in 12 weeks.

To take this test, you will need:

1. An adult friend.
2. A pillow.
3. A firm surface such as a kitchen counter or sturdy kitchen table.
4. An inexpensive Ace hardware or other hardware inclinometer.

Now you are ready to take the test.

Spine Strength Testing

A woman ideally should have 100 percent of her body weight as muscle strength in her back. Confused? Okay, what I mean is that if a woman weighs 120 pounds, then she should be able to use a Nautilus or Cybex low back machine and be able to push the bar weighted to 120 pounds for 10 repetitions.

A man has more muscle mass per pound of body weight and should be able to push 120 percent of his body weight on a similar machine. If he weighs 150 pounds, then 120 percent of 150 pounds is 150 x 1.20 = 180 pounds. He should be able to push 180 pounds 10 times.

If you don't have access to a back strengthening machine, then there is a home test that will give similar results. First, find a firm surface such as a counter that will allow you to lie on it with your body above the waist extended off the end of the counter. Have another adult lie across your legs so you don't fall. Place a pillow under your hips. Put your hands behind your neck. Bend all the way down so your upper body is at 90 degrees to your legs and then raise your trunk up again until it is in a straight line with your body. See illustrations 1 and 2.

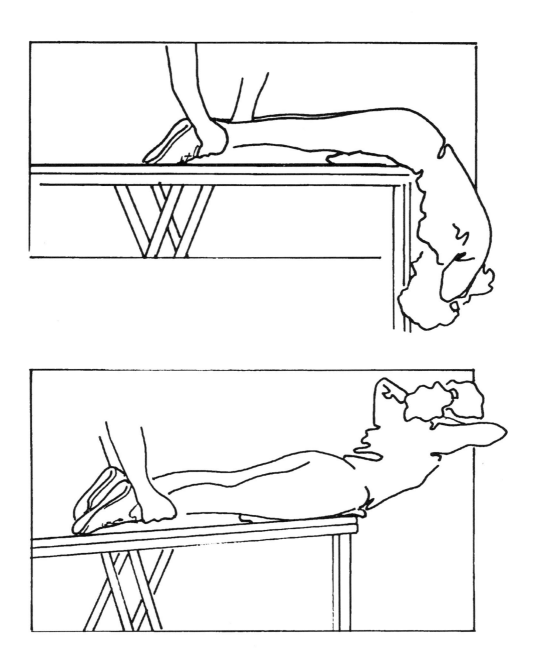

Illustrations 1 and 2

If you are a woman, you should be able to do this 10 times. If you are a man, you should be able to do this 12 times. Record the number in this space_____. If you can't do the exercise at all, then don't be discouraged. You have the most to gain from a program that restores function. If you are a woman taking the test, give yourself 10 points for each repetition. A man should give himself 8 1/2 points for each repetition. Write the total number of points out of a possible 100 points in the blank space in front of the words spine strength testing.

Following is a table for determining your strength based on the number of repetitions on the strength test.

Strength For Women		Strength For Men	
1 Repetition	10 Points	1 Repetition	8 Points
2 Repetitions	20 Points	2 Repetitions	16 Points
3 Repetitions	30 Points	3 Repetitions	25 Points
4 Repetitions	40 Points	4 Repetitions	33 Points
5 Repetitions	50 Points	5 Repetitions	41 Points
6 Repetitions	60 Points	6 Repetitions	50 Points
7 Repetitions	70 Points	7 Repetitions	58 Points
8 Repetitions	80 Points	8 Repetitions	66 Points
9 Repetitions	90 Points	9 Repetitions	75 Points
10 Repetitions	100 Points	10 Repetitions	83 Points
		11 Repetitions	91 Points
		12 Repetitions	100 Points

_____ Back Flexibility Testing

To perform this portion of the SAFE test accurately, you will need to purchase a protractor or inclinometer from your hardware store. In the example, we are using an inexpensive Ace Hardware inclinometer or protractor. See illustration 3.

Normal flexion of the spine is 72 degrees. In illustration 4, the middle of the inclinometer is placed approximately eight inches above the small of the back until it settles on zero degrees. Move it slightly up or down until it settles on zero degrees.

Have your partner or family member hold the meter in position while you keep your knees straight then bend forward as far as possible without pain. See illustrations 4 and 5. What you are measuring here is back and hip flexion. Since your starting number is 0 degrees and

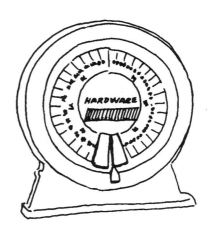

Illustration 3

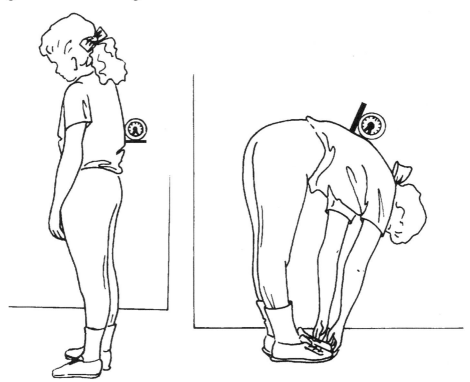

Illustrations 4 and 5

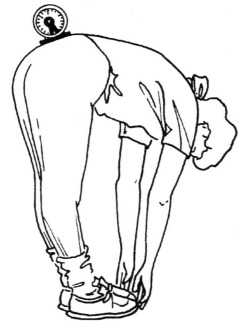

Illustration 6

your ending number is 75 degrees, you have a 75 degree difference between your ending number of 75 degrees and the starting number 0. Jot this number on the meter here_____.

The next thing you want to know is how much work your back performs when you bend forward and how much bending your hips are doing. To do this we measure hip motion.

Stand upright, then place the meter three inches below the belt line on the bony sacrum. Mark the number on the meter here ____. Then bend forward again as far as possible without pain and record that number here ____. Subtract the second number from the first number and record here ____. This is hip flexion. See illustration 6.

The formula is total back and hip flexion ____ minus hip flexion ____ equals back flexion ____. Write the number in the space in front of back flexibility testing. The rest are simpler to calculate.

_____Back Extension

Normally, both men and women have 45 degrees of backward bending or extension. To measure yours, place the meter about eight inches above the low back until it registers zero. Now bend as far backward as you can without bending your knees and have your partner record the number he sees on the meter attached to your back here_____. Subtract the ending number from the beginning number to get the total degrees of extension and write down that number in the space in front of the words back extension. See illustrations 7 and 8.

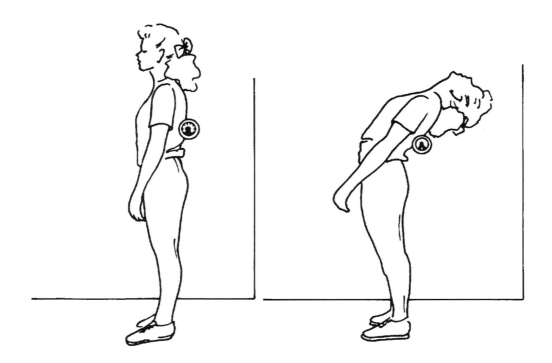

Illustrations 7 and 8

_____**Side Bending Right**

Place the meter eight inches above the small of your back as you see demonstrated in illustration 9. Line up the meter with zero degrees and then bend to the right. Record the degrees and place in front of the title side bending right.

_____**Side Bending Left**

Next bend to the left and record degrees that appear on the meter at the end of the movement. Mark this in front of side bending left.

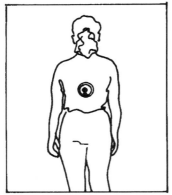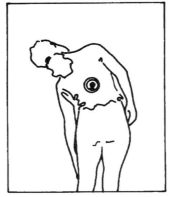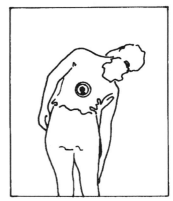

Illustrations 9, 10 and 11

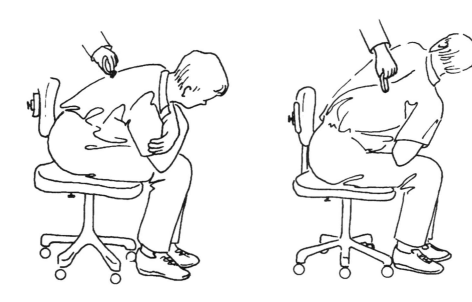

Illustrations 12 and 13

_____Rotating Right

Sit forward on a chair, then bend forward about 45 degrees. Set the inclinometer between the shoulder blades. Cross your hands and place the palms on the opposite shoulder. Slowly rotate to the right. Record the right rotation in the space in front of rotating right. For help, refer to Illustrations 12 and 13.

_____Rotating Left

Repeat the process to the left. Usually, one side of your body will be stiffer than the other. Record the left rotation in front of rotating left.

_____Straight Leg Raising Right

The test evaluates the flexibility of the hips and the hamstring muscles that assist the normal motion of your back. Start out by lying down on the floor. Lay the meter on the leg and knee until it registers zero. Then, keeping the knee straight, raise your right leg and foot as high as you can without using your hands to help. Record the number in the space in front of straight leg raising right. For help, refer to illustrations 14 and 15.

_____Straight Leg Raising Left

Repeat the test on the left leg and write the degrees in the space in front of straight leg raising left.

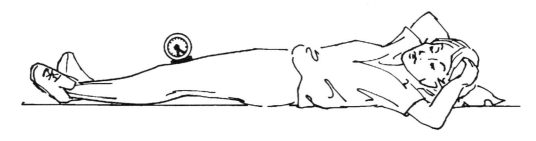

Illustration 14

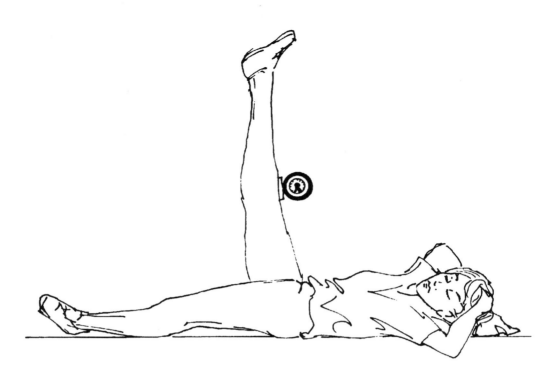

Illustration 15

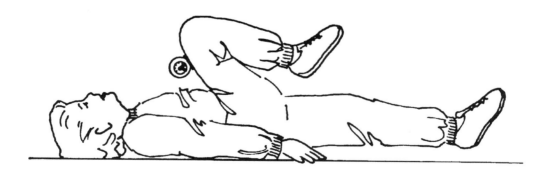

Illustration 16

_____Knee To Chest Right

This portion of the SAFE test measures the flexibility of the muscles that help to raise you to a standing position from a sitting position. In this case, set the meter on your right thigh and knee until it registers zero. Bend the knee up as close to the chest as possible without using your hands, Record the degrees in the space in front of knee to chest right. See illustration16.

_____Knee To Chest Left

Repeat this maneuver on the left side and record degrees in the space in front of knee to chest left.

LUMBAR SPINE FLEXIBILITY (Range Of Motion Measurements)

Look at your degrees of motion for each part of the test and circle your results on the sheet. Example, if you had 66 degrees of straight leg raising on the right side and 70 degrees on the left side, that would be six points on the right and seven points on the left side.

Straight Leg Raise (Record each Side)		Knee To Chest (Record each Side)	
Degrees	Points	Degrees	Points
100 +	10	130 +	10
90 - 99	9	115 - 129	9
80 - 89	8	100 - 114	8
70 - 79	7	85 - 99	7
60 - 69	6	70 - 84	6
50 - 59	5	55 - 69	5
40 - 49	4	40 - 54	4
30 - 39	3	25 - 39	3
20 - 29	2	15 - 24	2
10 - 19	1	5 - 14	1
Below 10	0	Below 5	0

Lumbar Flexion

Degrees	Points
75 +	10
68 - 74	9
60 - 67	8
53 - 59	7
46 - 52	6
39 - 45	5
32 - 38	4
25 - 31	3
18 - 24	2
11 - 17	1
Below 11	0

Lumbar Extension

Degrees	Points
30 +	10
27 - 29	9
24 - 26	8
21 - 23	7
18 - 20	6
15 - 17	5
12 - 14	4
9 - 11	3
6 - 8	2
3 - 5	1
Below 3	0

Side Bending
(Record for each Side)

Degrees	Points
30 +	10
27 - 29	9
24 - 26	8
21 - 23	7
18 - 20	6
15 - 17	5
12 - 14	4
9 - 11	3
6 - 8	2
3 - 5	1
Below 3	0

Rotation
(Record for each Side)

Degrees	Points
30 +	10
27 - 29	9
24 - 26	8
21 - 23	7
18 - 20	6
15 - 17	5
12 - 14	4
9 - 11	3
6 - 8	2
3 - 5	1
Below 3	0

ENDURANCE TESTING

Muscle endurance is important because it is a measure of strength plus contraction time. If your muscles are very weak, your endurance will be low initially.

_____**Upper Abdomen Muscles**

Lie on your back on the floor with your knees bent. See illustration 17. Ask your partner to hold your feet. Place your hands behind your neck. Do a partial sit up until your shoulder blades are off the floor and hold for up to

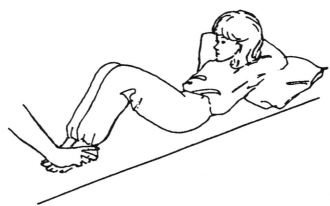

Illustration 17

20 seconds. You will feel tension in your abdomen and tightness. Record the number of seconds in the space in front of upper abdomen muscles.

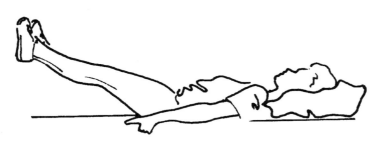

Illustration 18

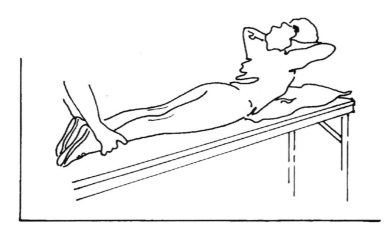

_____Lower Abdomen Muscles

Lie on your back with a pillow behind your neck and raise both legs up to a 45 degree position. Hold for up to 20 seconds. Record your seconds in the space in front of lower abdomen muscles.

Illustration 19

_____Upper Lumbar Muscles

Lie on your stomach as indicated in illustration 19 while your assistant holds your feet on the floor. Put your hands behind your neck. Now raise up until your chest is at least four inches off the floor. Hold this for up to 20 seconds. Record your seconds in the space in front of upper lumbar muscles.

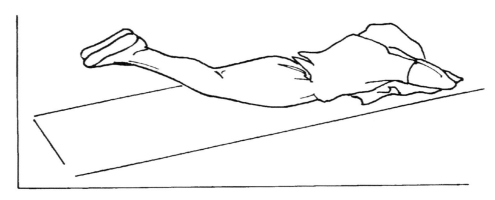

Illustration 20

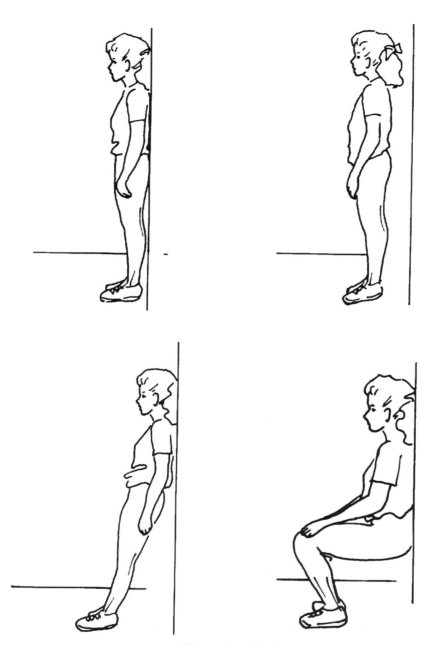

Illustrations 21 through 24

_____Lower Lumbar Muscles

Lie on your stomach on the floor. Put your hands under your forehead and raise both feet off the floor 6 inches, hold for up to 20 seconds. See illustration 20. Record the number of seconds in the space in front of lower lumbar muscles.

_____Quadriceps or Thigh Strength

Stand with your back against a wall. Take one step forward. Now squat while your back slides down against the wall. When your thighs are parallel with the floor, hold for up to 20 seconds. See illustrations 21 through 24. Record the total number of seconds in front of quadriceps strength.

Now, record your total number of endurance points here_____vs 100.

AEROBIC PROGRAM

The aerobic program is based on research that indicates oxygen and nutrients are delivered by this form of exercise. They are necessary for new muscle growth and for optimum performance of your back. I've chosen five categories of aerobic fitness to use as standards. Select one of these five to perform without undue stress on your body. Later on, after you've conditioned your body with the exercise described in the book, you'll discover you have raised your level of aerobic fitness.

Each level represents a specific amount of oxygen "burned" by your body. Ask your physician for permission to perform the aerobics you select before your begin. The symbol ml/Kg/minute means that your body uses so many milliliters of oxygen per kilogram of body weight per minute. In this test you only need to know the points you generate. This test shows how efficiently your cardiovascular system performs. These levels do not challenge "elite" athletes, but evaluate the aerobic condition of the aspiring health-conscious individual.

<u>100 Points Utilizes 35 ml/Kg/Minute of Oxygen</u>
>Run one mile in less than eight minutes or
>Bicycle five miles in less than 20 minutes or
>Run in place for 12 1/2 minutes. *Run at 80/90 steps/minute.

<u>80 Points Utilizes 28 ml/Kg/Minute of Oxygen</u>
>Run one mile in less than 10 minutes or
>Bicycle four miles in less than 24 minutes or
>Run in place for 10 minutes. *Run at 80/90 steps/minute.

<u>60 Points Utilizes 21ml/Kg/Minute of Oxygen</u>
>Run or walk one mile in less than 12 minutes or
>Bicycle three miles in less than 12 minutes or
>Run in place for 7 1/2 minutes. *Run at 80/90 steps/minute.

<u>40 Points Utilizes 14 ml/Kg/Minute of Oxygen</u>
>Run or walk one mile in less than 14 minutes or
>Bicycle two miles in less than 8 minutes or
>Run in place for 5 minutes. *Run at 80/90 steps/minute.

<u>20 Points Utilizes 7ml/Kg/Minute of Oxygen</u>
>Run or walk one mile in 16 minutes or
>Bicycle two miles in 12 minutes
>Run in place for 2-1/2 minutes. *Run at 80/90 steps/minute.

Circle The Number Of Points You Have Earned
In The Aerobic Program

Comment: After a back injury, many people are unable to run on a hard surface but some can tolerate running on a soft, grassy surface, a small trampoline or rubberized track like those found at many high schools. Various options are offered to provide you with choices to test your aerobic conditioning. Frequently after back pain develops, these activities are discontinued with the result that you may not even make the fifth category of

7ml/Kg/minute of oxygen utilized. In a short time, with effort you will move up from one category to another. Don't be discouraged by your performance on any of these tests. They are given only to provide you with an idea of the condition of your body and back in relation to what it can be with some effort. By repeating the test every four weeks, you will be able to watch your progress.

RECORD YOUR ENDURANCE POINTS

Upper Abdomen. Give yourself one point for each second you held this position. Maximum points you can earn is 20. Record here_____.

Lower Abdomen. Give yourself one point for every second you held this position. Maximum points you can earn is 20. Record here_____.

Upper Lumbar. Give yourself one point for every second you held this position. Maximum points you can earn is 20. Record here_____.

Lower Lumbar. Give yourself one point for every second you held this position. Maximum points you can earn is 20. Record here_____.

Quadriceps Strength. Give yourself 20 points for every second you held this position. Maximum points you can earn is 20. Record here_____.

RECORD YOUR TOTAL POINTS ON THE SAFE TEST

Total Strength Points   _____
Total Aerobic Points   _____
Total Flexibility Points   _____
Total Endurance Points   _____

Add all four numbers and divide by four for the average. This is your healthy back index score on the SAFE Test.

HEALTHY BACK INDEX

91-100 Points	Great! You did it. You have a healthy back!
81-90 Points	Do the 10-minute exercises to stay in shape.
61-80 Points	Good, you need four weeks in the program.
41-60 Points	Poor. Three months will change your shape and the way you feel.
21-40 Points	You feel aged beyond your years. You will be able to restore function in four months. Don't give up, you have the most to gain.

For most individuals it takes one month on this program to reach the next level of the HEALTHY BACK INDEX. Even if you have only 15 points, you can restore health to your back. With only 15 points, it will take about four months. Don't be frustrated by this score, the four months are going to pass whether or not you begin the program. Where do you begin? See Chapter 9, *Armor-Plating The Spine*. See Chapter 10, *Building Endurance and Performance*, and see Chapter 11 for *Stretching* which restores flexibility.

PROGRESS CHART OF BACK TEST RESULTS

	Date	Points
Spine Strength Testing	_____	_____
Flexibility Testing		
Back flexion	_____	_____
Back extension	_____	_____
Side bending right	_____	_____
Side bending left	_____	_____
Rotation right	_____	_____
Rotation left	_____	_____
Straight leg raise right	_____	_____
Straight leg raise left	_____	_____
Knee to chest right	_____	_____
Knee to chest left	_____	_____
Total Flexibility Points	_____	_____
Endurance Testing		
Upper abdomen	_____	_____
Lower abdomen	_____	_____
Upper lumbar	_____	_____
Lower lumbar	_____	_____
Quadriceps	_____	_____
Total Endurance Points	_____	_____
Total Aerobic Points	_____	_____

Total Spine Strength _____ +
Aerobic Points _____ +
Flexibility _____ +
Endurance _____ =
_____ Divide by 4 for Score _____

< 3 >

Well-defined Backs Are Built, Not Born

Exercise ten minutes a day
to offset office fatigue and tone muscles.

Please examine the drawing of the musculature of the torso shown on page 30. It will help you to understand why muscles must be kept in good condition. They protect the spine, keeping it firm and healthy.

Remember, a healthy back stays that way from a supporting cast of strong and flexible muscles. That's why the simple routine on the following pages zeroes in on key back-stabilizing muscles in the torso and the legs. It specifically stretches the flexors, muscles in the front of the body that tend to get tight and short without enough use, and strengthens the extensors—the muscles in the back that weaken with underuse. The exercises also bolster the spine-supporting abdominals. Results: Backache prevention and relief and a trimmer middle and straighter posture.

Well-defined backs are built not born. Practice three of the exercises shown every day, for 10 minutes. Rotate the exercises so that in a four-day period, you will practice each one of them. They are designed to offset office fatigue and build muscle elasticity and endurance. They will strengthen crucial back sections with weights, bars, and Thera-Bands. Choose a resistance that allows you to do at least 10, but no more than 15 repetitions.

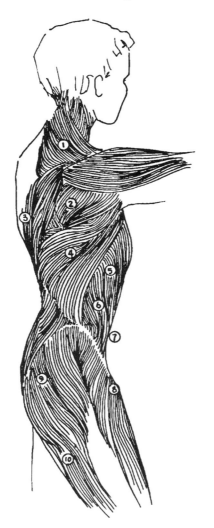

THE MUSCLES SUPPORTING THE BACK
(Abdominals)

While back pain shows up in the spine, it is the muscles supporting the spine that keep you free of pain.

These are: The trapezius (1), deep shoulder muscles (2), and paraspinal (3). Underneath the trapezius are muscles that require strength and stretching to support the posture of the spine (4). Strong abdominals—the oblique muscles (5), the transversus (6), and rectus abdominus (7)—eliminate stress on the lower back. Supple psoas muscles (8) and other interior muscles (not visible)—or hip flexors help maintain youthful movement and agility, while strong glutei maximi (9) provide back protection and balance. A post-exercise cool down should always include plenty of hamstring (10) stretching.

REAR-LAT PULLDOWN
(Latissimus dorsi)

Stand, hold ends of Thera-Band, and extend arms overhead. (For comfort, wrap bands around knuckles and fingers.) Slowly bring arms down and behind the head, keeping them wide for resistance. Bring arms up slowly and repeat. (In the weight room, for those seated, using a high pulley with a wide grip bar.) Start withband in front of shoulders, then move upward and over shoulders toward the back.

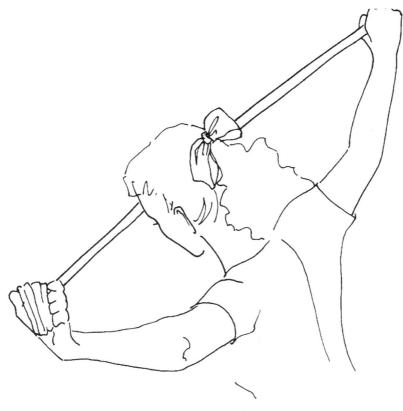

Illustration 26

ABDOMINAL CRUNCH
(Abdominals)

Lie on your back with legs up and bent slightly, feet crossed and hands behind your head. Contracting abdominals pressing lower back into floor, slowly raise your head and shoulders. Release slightly and repeat contractions in a pulsing action, 10 to 15 times. Add a twist to each side for 10 to 15 repetitions.

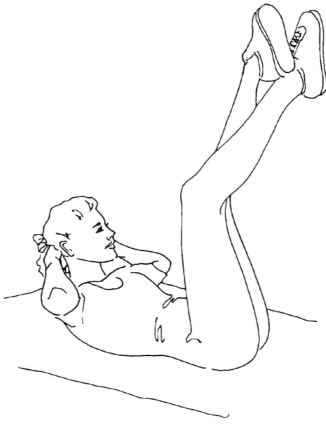

Illustration 27

YOGA TWIST
(Paraspinal and lower muscles)

Seated, extend the right leg and cross the left over it, holding the left knee back with the right arm, twisting around with the head and upper body and looking left. Hold for at least 15 seconds, release and switch sides.

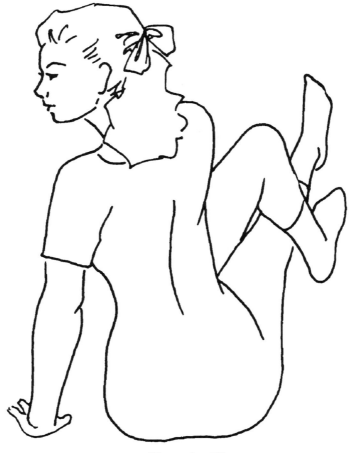

Illustration 28

CAT BACK
(Paraspinal and lower back)

On hands and knees, head level to spine, round back by pulling the abdominal muscles toward the ceiling, then reverse neutral position: imagine a cat stretching. Repeat three times.

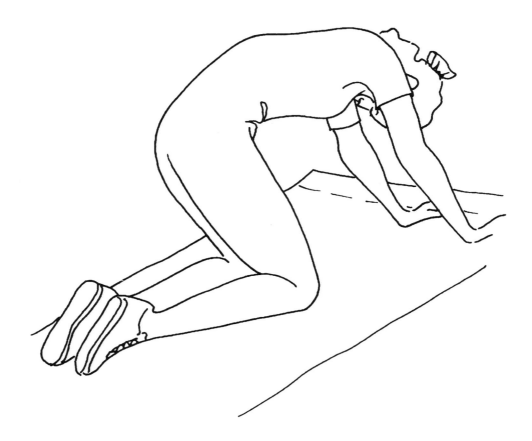

Illustration 29

ROUND THE CLOCK
(Lower back)

Lie on your back holding knees to chest. Slowly circle knees as if moving around a clock, feeling the lumbar region (lower back) press to the floor. Reverse.

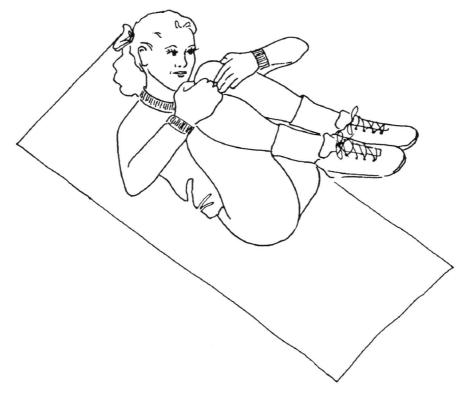

Illustration 30

SPHINX
(Abdominal muscles and lower back)

Lie on stomach, elbows under shoulders. Slowly press up, keeping stomach muscles firm and without straining back. Come up to forearms, hold for 10 seconds, release down. Repeat three times.

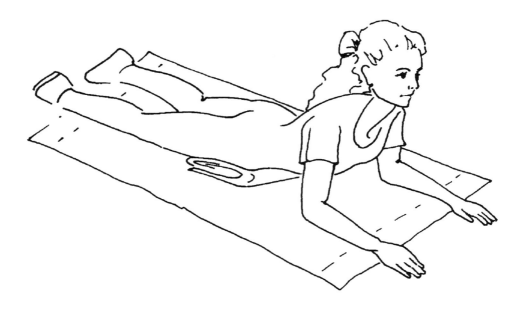

Illustration 31

HIP FLEXION
(Thighs and hips)

Lie on your back on a bench or table. Bring right knee into chest. Hold for at least 15 seconds, breathing deeply. Repeat with left leg.

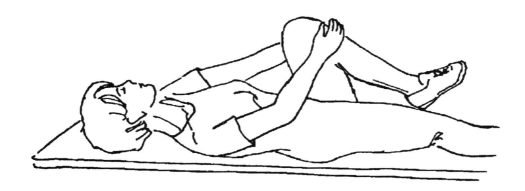

Illustration 32

BACK-LATERAL RAISE
(Trapezius, paraspinal, rhomboids)

Sit at the end of a bench resting chest on thighs, with dumbells close to your feet. Pick up the weights, then slowly raise them out to the side, as shown, keeping elbows slightly bent and squeezing shoulder blades together. Keep the back flat. Lower and repeat.

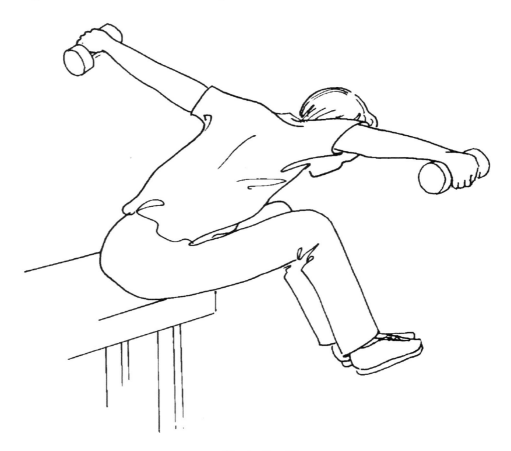

Illustration 33

SEATED ROW
(Lats, rhomboids, paraspinals)

Sit with right leg extended, left leg bent, Thera-Band around right foot held with one end in each hand. Keeping chest lifted, shoulders down and elbows in, pull back as far as possible, as shown. Hold, then release and slowly repeat. (In weight room use a low pulley.)

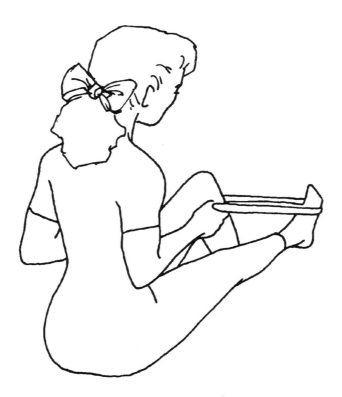

Illustration 34

SINGLE-ARM ROW
(Lats, trapezius)

Place dumbells on the floor, then with right hand and knee on the bench, and keeping your back flat, abdominals in, reach down and slowly bring the weight up beside your ribs. Lower and repeat. Change arms after each set.

Illustration 35

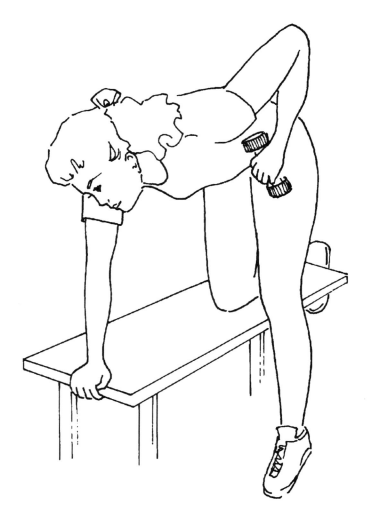

BENT-OVER ROW
(Lats, trapezius, paraspinal muscles)

Place weighted bar with or without weights on the floor. Bend forward from the hips, keeping knees slightly bent, chest forward, abdominals in and back flat. Raise the bar, bringing it up until it touches your chest lightly. Lower slowly and repeat.

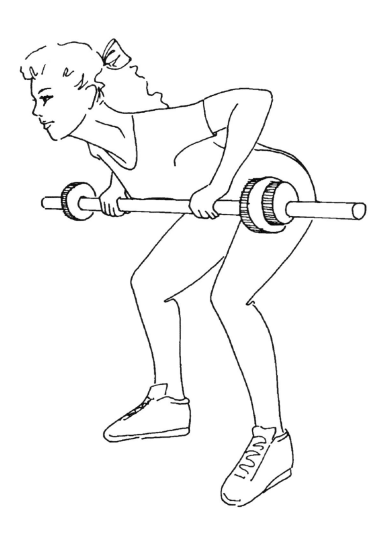

Illustration 36

< 4 >

Four Out Of Five Of Us Will Experience
Back Trouble

*Physical neglect is the prime reason
people see a physician or chiropractor.*

Nothing can make you feel old and vulnerable more quickly than a sudden back attack. One moment you are doing a routine chore and the next you are astonished by a pain in your back that takes your breath away.

If you've been surprised by a bad back, it's probably little comfort to know that four out of five adults will share your experience at some period in their lives. If the Eighties was the decade of heart and health awareness, then the Nineties will surely be the years of emphasis on the back as the population of baby-boomers reaches the critical age—from 30 to 55—when back problems strike.

Yet, only a small percentage of back problems are really serious. Simple muscle strain—resulting from physical neglect—is the primary reason 80 percent of us will see a doctor or chiropractor for back pain in our life times. Unfortunately, many of us never resume normal activities again because many physicians do not themselves understand how the back works and how to keep it healthy.

As I said earlier, the most commonly prescribed treatment for back pain, "rest therapy", which often puts a person in bed for days or weeks, is the worst advice that can be given for back strain. Inactive people "resting" their backs, waiting for the pain to subside, lose muscle strength at a rate of three percent of the total muscle mass for every day of idleness. By the time the pain is gone and the patient cautiously resumes physical activity, his back is weaker than it was prior to the strain and is more vulnerable to a new injury. Millions of Americans suffer from back weakness, muscle softness and physical disability as the result of medical advice that encourages this lack of activity.

The cause of back pain, more often than not, is years of bad back habits. So what can you do to buck the odds? How can you prepare your back to prevent injury and pain and impaired quality of life?

Avoidance of bad habits is the answer. A little daily attention at home and at work can keep your back young for a long, long time.

By following the simple exercises demonstrated in this book, you can not only prevent back problems from developing, but you can rehabilitate an injured back. Such is the inherent ability of the back to restore itself, rejuvenate weak muscle, grow vital tissues and toughen bones, that even people over 90 years old can bring new vigor to their aging backs and increase their muscle strength by 300 percent in just twelve weeks. If the elderly—people who have actually become stiff, brittle and cramped as the result of inactivity and aging—can develop healthy backs, clearly young and middle-aged people can become free of back pain. The exercises demonstrated in *Back Works* are designed to rehabilitate and strengthen out-of-condition backs and armor-plate them so they will be almost impervious to ordinary stresses and strains.

Ordinary stresses and strains are the major causes of back injuries.

The simple act of stretching to remove a bag of groceries from the trunk of a car can cause strain that can incapacitate you if you have a soft back and keep you in pain for days or weeks. "Rest" therapy not only worsens the injury but increases the chances of re-injury. And once a back injury occurs, the chances of it happening again are four times more likely than if you had kept your back active in the first place. Staying in shape with simple, but effective exercises, improves the blood flow essential for the spine's health and builds strong, flexible muscles to protect the spine.

LOW BACK PAIN RELATED TO TRAUMA

Who gets back pain? What causes it? Let's view the back for answers. The back is an engineering puzzle that can withstand the crush of a tackle by a 300 pound lineman, yet it may "slip out of place" when you bend over to pick up a sock.

To start, we need a basic idea of how the spine works. Look at illustration 37. The picture on the left is the side view of the spine. As you can see, the spine is made up of curves to help absorb the shock of daily activities. In the lower portion of the spine a circle has been drawn to illustrate one functional unit of the spine. A functional unit contains one vertebra, such as the third lumbar vertebra or L3, along with the disc and vertebra above and below.

On the large close up view, the vertebral "blocks" are separated by cushions or discs that change shape when, for example, you stand while holding a weight or while bending backwards.

In a side view of the spine, illustration 38, a disc is shown, located between the L3 and L4 vertebrae which herniates or pushes out backwards into the spinal canal against the spinal nerves. At this level the spinal nerves run into the legs and a disc herniation in this location will usually produce leg and buttock pain.

Pain also can be caused by abnormal motion between the vertebrae due to muscle weakness. If you experience back pain from bending forward, the tendency is to avoid the activity that causes the pain. As a result, the

Side View of the Spine

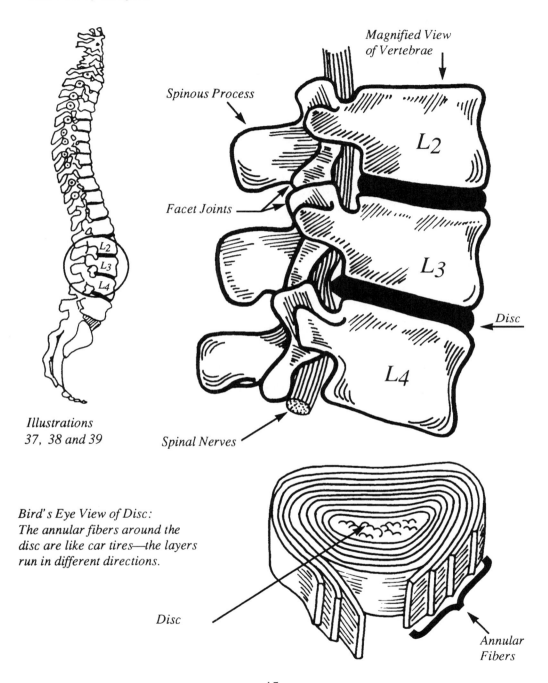

Magnified View of Vertebrae

Spinous Process

Facet Joints

L2

L3

Disc

L4

Spinal Nerves

Illustrations 37, 38 and 39

Bird's Eye View of Disc: The annular fibers around the disc are like car tires—the layers run in different directions.

Disc

Annular Fibers

muscles become tight, stiff and more painful. Muscles act like guy wires that support a tall radio tower. They maintain the spine in proper position and assist us in our daily living activities. Just as guy wires require preventative maintenance, so do your back muscles. If you don't keep them in shape, you may hear from your back in a painful way.

Dark black lines represent minor tears or injuries that are cumulative. Concentric rings are protective annular fibers.

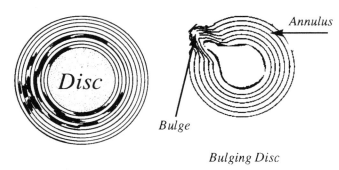

Bulging Disc

Illustration 40

Most books about back pain incorrectly describe the discs between the vertebrae as a "jelly donut." When you injure the donut, the "jelly" pushes out backward. If a disc really were like jelly, it wouldn't hurt when it ruptured. The fact is, the disc is the middle or central part of the area between each vertebra. In reality, the outer layers of the disc area are like car tires. They run in several different directions and there are several layers. See illustration 40. When the disc and its outer protective layers are damaged, the blood supply to the disc is decreased and it changes composition "drying out" from soft material to firm or hard material. As additional minor injuries or strains produce more damage, the disc hardens and may push through torn layers of the protective annulus fibers. See illustration 40. If it pushes out too far, then the disc ruptures and may press on the spinal nerves resulting in severe leg pain, back pain or both.

What happens if you strain your back or "pull a muscle?" While the affected muscle will heal in three to six weeks, the muscles around it go into spasm immediately. The spasm acts like a splint to hold the injured muscle in the correct position while it heals. Often the body overreacts to protect the injured muscle and causes too much spasming which you feel as a painful "grabbing" sensation in your back. In order to restore the muscles, they need to be gently stretched and worked to prevent tight, stiff scar tissue from forming in the area.

Every bone or vertebra in the spine is held in alignment with its neighbors by ligaments—white, tough connective tissue. When ligaments are torn, they heal poorly due to depleted blood supply. If you have many damaged ligaments, you have an unstable low back or one that may "clunk" or "thunk" and give you sharp pain when you are involved in certain activities.

What if an injury involving ligaments and a disc doesn't heal? Do you need surgery? Not usually. A program aimed at restoring function to your spine by restoring strength and flexibility will transfer most of the movements of the ligament and disc to muscles. You can actually measure how much exercise you need to perform for your muscles to work at their best.

While the discs and muscles are two major areas of pain-causing problems, a third one is the joints between the vertebrae. These are called

Bird's Eye View Of Disk And Spine Segment

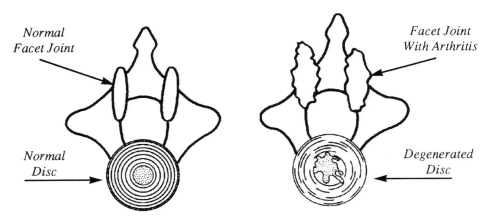

Normal Facet Joint

Facet Joint With Arthritis

Normal Disc

Degenerated Disc

Illustration 41

— 47 —

facet (fuh-set´) joints and they connect the back of the upper vertebrae to the back of the lower vertebrae. They guide the movement of the spine and allow you to bend forward and backward as the facets slide across one another. See illustration 41.

Among the other main causes of back pain are poor posture, and walking with the shoulders stooped or with weak or flabby abdominal muscles—a pot belly. See illustration 42. A pot belly frequently brings on back pain by forcing the person to bend backward while walking, putting pressure on the small facet joints which are too small to bear the weight of an obese body. Actually, the weight of a pot belly pulls the back into an abnormally shaped curve which can pinch or irritate small spinal nerves and cause pain.

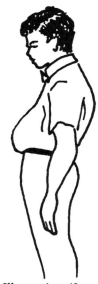

Illustration 42

Osteoarthritis, the wear-and-tear arthritis that most of us experience as part of the aging process, is another cause of back pain. But it isn't a hard and fast rule that if you have arthritis you will have pain.

Stress and worry cause back pain. Concerns about money, family, jobs, may keep your back in a constant state of spasm as you fret and make adrenaline in response to stress. Adrenaline causes the muscles to tense as part of the fight or flight mechanism in all humans.

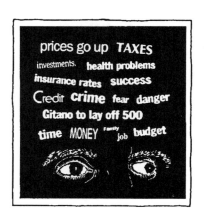

There are unusual causes of back pain that are created by birth defects. Also, spinal curvatures can cause pain as can some pelvic or prostate problems.

A cause of back pain not originating in the back happens when

If the hamstring muscle does not stretch with bending then the lower back has to do more of the bending and becomes at risk of injury. Hamstring muscle is crosshatched in drawings

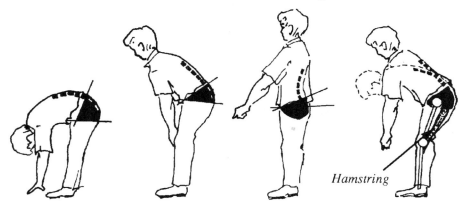

Hamstring

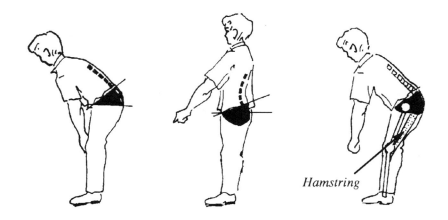

Hamstring

Illustration 44

hamstring muscles in the legs are tight. See illustration 44. Tight hamstring muscles—often resulting from lack of exercise and stretching—prevent the pelvis from bending forward when you bend over. The result is that the lumbar spine may have to perform twice as much movement as normal, causing back pain. This is especially true for a person who is lifting while bending.

LOW BACK PAIN RELATED TO TRAUMA

Major trauma and what may seem to be insignificant insults to the low back can result in severe disability. The following stories are offered to show the reader how different people handled their crises. How any person responds to injury is an indication of his motivation, personality and drive to succeed. These narratives of back injury may help you to understand how versatile the human back is and how exercise treatment can help restore function to it.

Compression Injury

To Devon the whine of the engines, the smell of hot steel were like a bracing tonic. He looked around at busy workers hurrying in all directions as forklifts and cranes carried materials to men at stations in the foundry. Casting metal parts was Devon's specialty. He was an artist at turning molten steel and aluminum into useable shapes. One day he would be the engineer who created the designs of steel parts. He had completed one year of college and was going to night school four days each week to get his degree.

This week he was casting high-performance aluminum engine blocks to be used in an Indy race car. He wanted to do the clean up of these newly-cast blocks, a job he normally disliked. But in this case, he felt like the motor blocks were pieces of auto sports history in the making.

Because the soft metal scratched and dented more easily than steel, the crane used to lift them was fitted with a padded cradle to carry each finished motor block to quality control. There the cylinders in each block would be

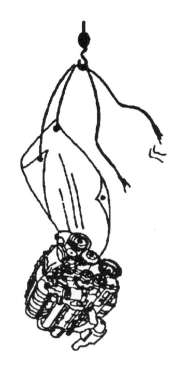

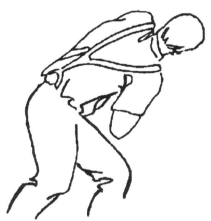

Illustration 45

measured for the correct tolerances.

As each new engine block moved down the line between rows of men, Devon walked alongside. He stepped ahead of one swinging block and cradle to signal a forklift driver when, suddenly, the cable snapped on the cradle. The forward momentum of the engine carried it in a descending arc toward Devon. It was already too late when he heard the cable snap and turned his head to look over his shoulder. The engine block struck Devon directly in the center of his low back knocking him off his feet and pinning him to the floor. He could not move his legs or even feel them. Sirens wailed as all activity in the foundry stopped. Emergency medical technicians arrived on the scene to transport Devon to the hospital.

Devon was rushed into surgery. The weight and momentum of the aluminum engine block had crushed a disc in his lower back and caused a rupture of his spleen in the abdomen. He was bleeding internally so profusely that his spleen had to be removed.

After surgery, Devon could feel his legs again. His doctor told him that initially he had suffered spinal cord shock that temporarily caused the loss of all sensation in his back and use of his legs. After recuperating for six weeks, Devon wanted to return to work but was unable to because of low back pain. He was told that he might never be able to return to his job again because of the permanent damage to the disc between lumbar 4 and lumbar 5 vertebra. This was because the blow from the engine block ruptured a disc in his back forcing it upward into the bone of the vertebra above, resulting in significant pain. The shock to his spinal cord was a result of swelling around the cord and spasm of the blood vessels that supplied blood to the cord. See illustration 46.

Side View - Devon's Injury

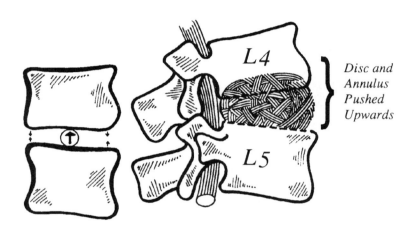

Illustration 46

Devon refused to accept the idea that he would have to be an invalid. He was not about to sit home and receive disability checks. He rarely sat down to watch television. He was action oriented and was determined to prove the doctors wrong.

While the disc in his back was partially crushed and painful, it did not require surgery and would not result in any paralysis. He learned that with an injured disc the back's function can be restored through a program aimed at slowly increasing the mobility of each part of the lower back, including strengthening exercises of the lumbar muscles.

Devon approached rehabilitation like an Olympic athlete. He was focused on the single purpose of increasing his strength and flexibility. He worked slowly and thoroughly at the task of building muscles. When, later, he returned to work, he still experienced some pain, but was able to perform his job and finish school. He now is a "working" engineer who is not content to sit in an office and design metal products. He is a team leader and sets the example for six co-workers in the development and production of metal alloy parts.

If you have been injured and want to return to work, there is a job out there for you. If you have trouble finding it, then vocational rehabilitation specialists will help you. Ask your doctor or claims examiner for the name of one of these counselors.

Low Back Strain and Sprain

The simple task of lifting a bag of groceries out of his car laid Jim Davidson low. A streak of pain shot across his lower back so unexpectedly that it took his breath away. He was bedridden for three weeks, nursing his back, moving cautiously to avoid jabbing attacks of pain. He had decided that he would not see a doctor. *Incompetents! Charlatans!* They had taken his mother's money, but had never been able to help her back. As he looked up at the ceiling in his bedroom, Jim thought about his mother. A forlorn back cripple, she had spent most of her days in bed or on the sofa suffering mutely with determined anguish.

Jim vowed to himself that he would never end up as his mother had. That meant he had to do something for himself. Slowly, he formulated a plan then climbed carefully out of bed and dressed, his anxious movements like those of a frail old man. He had made the decision to take charge of his back and his life.

On the first day of his recuperation, Jim hobbled out to the mailbox. His face broke out in a sweat and his legs shook but he made it. The next day he walked to the end of the block. After two weeks, he was able to walk a

A Tear Of The Low Back Muscles
Jim's Injury

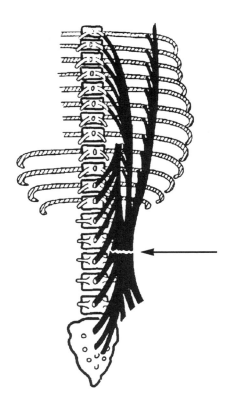

Illustration 47

mile. He still was unable to return to work.

Next, Jim joined Unlimited Fitness, a local health club. Although he couldn't lift any weights, he watched other members do stretches and copied them. The more he stretched, the better he felt and the less pain he had. He spent an hour stretching twice daily.

With the stretches helping to control the pain, he started lifting five-pound weights. Soon he moved up to 10 and then 20 pounds. He felt encouraged by his progress and cautiously started using weight lifting machines. After two weeks of lifting he was able to return to light-duty work. In a few months, Jim was in better physical condition than he had ever been in his life. He wasn't sure what to do next so he rode the exercycles and walked on the stair machine.

The low back machine was Jim's next target. He discovered that his pain increased as he exerted himself pushing against the bar. He stopped and stretched and repeated the process. After 20 minutes, he was delighted to find out that he could push the bar all the way back one time. Persisting, he worked at another repetition and another until his back muscles were too fatigued to perform.

In the next few weeks of working on the low back machine, Jim realized that while he felt better as a whole and was stronger, his back was still weak. He put more time on low back exercises. He augmented the machine with one hour of stretches in the morning and evening.

As time went on Jim became busier at his job and decreased his stretching time. One morning he awoke with the familiar pain in his back and he decided that he had to get back on his program again.

Why did the pain return when Jim reduced his strengthening and flexibility program? The answer is that when muscles have been injured, some of them or parts of them may have received permanent injury. Other close muscles can help to compensate for the weakness if they are strengthened. Muscles respond to use. Use a muscle and it gets stronger. Stop using it and it gets weaker. Weaker muscles do not give the back the stability it needs to perform the functions of bending, twisting and lifting. To maintain strength and flexibility an injured person like Jim needs to continue on a program. Rarely, however, does anyone need the kind of program as time-consuming as Jim's. Had Jim sought the advice of a rehabilitation expert he would have been directed to a program of muscle recovery more specific to his condition. He would have saved a lot of time—and pain.

"I'll Start My New Diet Tomorrow."

"Just one more bowl of potato chips and I'll stop snacking," vowed Mary Kay. Settled back into her favorite chair and armed with the current issue of TV Guide, Mary Kay controlled her environment from her central position between the kitchen, living room and dining room. She kept fresh batteries in the drawer of her end table for replacing the used ones in her TV remote control. Her children were used to getting more snacks for her during every commercial or bringing the newspaper or a magazine at her request.

Anyone who suffers as much as I do from back pain deserves to have people wait on them, she thought.

Mary Kay's back pain was the result of her obesity. The constant pressure of her weight on the discs of her low back caused nerves to twinge.

Mary Kay blamed her back problems and her extra 100 pounds on her back. Her fat was the result of inactivity brought on by her pain, she thought.

She was never aware of how her appearance affected her children until the Christmas show at the elementary school. Two days earlier she had joined other parents and grandparents eager to watch their small fry singing in the holiday spirit. Having arrived a few minutes late, Mary Kay entered the second to last row in the auditorium seeking a seat half way down the aisle. After climbing over six or seven people, she squirmed her way to her seat. With a sigh of relief, she plopped down on the metal chair and heard a horrible sound of crumbling steel. The old folding chair expired under her weight and came crashing to the floor. The commotion stilled the young singers on the stage and all eyes focused on Mary Kay. It seemed an eternity before she was able to extricate herself from the bent steel and make an escape. Her face continued to flush as she headed for the door with all eyes upon her. As she reached the outer doors of the grade school she heard the start-up of tiny voices half-singing and half-laughing—at her.

Marie, Mary Kay's young daughter was in tears and refused to attend school for two days after the incident. She refused to be seen shopping with her mother or anywhere in public.

Heart-broken over her daughter's embarrassment, Mary Kay decided to change her eating habits—the very next day.

Tomorrow came and Mary Kay went to a bookstore to find books on dieting and weight loss, asking the store manager for recommendations. At home, she read the books she had purchased, dipping pretzels into peanut butter and thinking she should eat healthier foods. When she discovered a section in one of her books entitled "Hidden Fats," she realized that her diet was 80-90 percent fat. The salads she ate when she was with her friends were piled high with oily dressings.

"Maybe I can cut my fat intake to 50 percent with a few changes in my snacks," she thought.

On her new regime, Mary Kay kept her pretzels, eating them without peanut butter and replaced cream-filled and chocolate-filled cookies with graham crackers. With only small changes in her diet she was able to lose five pounds for each of the first two weeks, then her weight loss slowed.

Back to the bookstore for more ideas. Mixed in with the books on self-improvement and diet was a book on diet and exercise. The thought of working up a sweat in a gym surrounded by muscular men or slim aerobic dancers was too embarrassing for Mary Kay. The book suggested she start walking. She began with five blocks daily and every three days added another block.

At the end of two months she was walking approximately two and one half miles per day and had lost an average of two pounds per week for 16 more pounds. Now, she had reduced her weight by 26 pounds. She was feeling much better, her buttons no longer pulled and gaped across her breasts and abdomen. Her shoe size went down from a ten to an eight as she continued to walk. An hour a day seemed like a long time but Mary Kay remembered the look on her daughter's face the day of the Christmas show.

As the months passed, Mary Kay studied labels when she shopped. She cut up her old size 15-1/2 smocks, able to get into size 14. Her weight stabilized at 150 pounds and she felt great. At 5'8", she received compliments about her new appearance and often was not recognized by people who had not seen her for months.

Mary Kay cut and pasted, borrowed and begged everything she could find on nutrition. On page 54 are 10 tips Mary Kay used for losing the fat that held her prisoner.

As Mary Kay discovered, walking helps to lose weight while at the same time it strengthens the low back. Each time you raise one foot to step forward, the low back muscles contract to stabilize your hips and pelvis from moving excessively up and down. As Mary Kay lost weight and exercised, her body responded.

It was not until a year after the Christmas show that she decided to join an indoor tennis club since the eastern Oregon winters can be difficult for a walking program. Mary Kay did poorly at tennis. She knew her back was stronger and she was breathing easily but her back was stiff from not stretching and she was unable to reach the "hard ones." Her serve was more difficult than she remembered from high school.

By now Mary Kay was practicing three of the four cornerstones of a healthy back. She had back strength and muscular endurance from hour long walks, and she was aerobically fit. She came to my office to find the missing link—flexibility. Measurements showed her to be at 44 percent of normal spine flexibility. We prescribed the knee to chest stretch, illustration 48, the back hyperextension, illustration 49, and the helicopter, illustration 50. With these three stretches and her already excellent program, Mary Kay was able to excel at athletic activities.

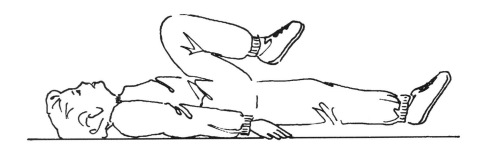

Illustration 48

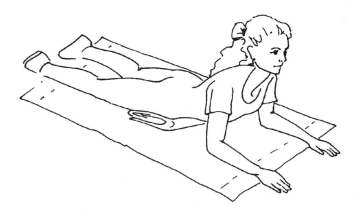

Illustration 49

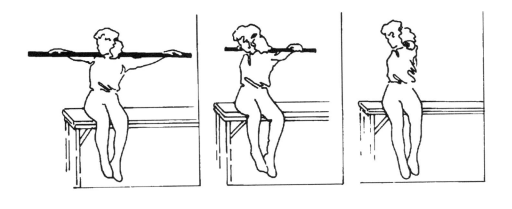

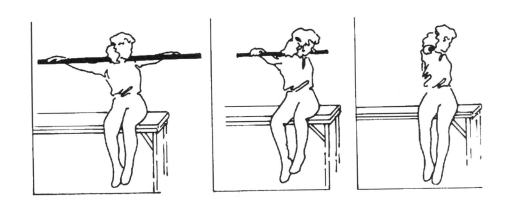

Illustration 50

Here are Mary Kay's 10 tips for losing fat:

1. Use the 944 Emergency Fat Rule. Fat contains 9 calories for each gram of fat. Carbohydrates and Protein each contain 4 calories for each gram of fat. As an example, 2% milk contains 37 percent fat calories. Here is the label of 2% milk:

```
┌─────────────────────────────────────────────────┐
│  NUTRITIONAL INFORMATION PER SERVING:            │
│                                                  │
│  Serving size .............................. 1 cup │
│  Servings per container ...................... 8 │
│  Calories .................................. 120 │
│  Protein ................................ 8 grams │
│  Carbohydrate ......................... 11 grams │
│  Fat ..................................... 5 grams │
│                                                  │
└─────────────────────────────────────────────────┘
```

Calculate protein calories. Eight grams times four calories per gram equals 32 calories. Then multiply carbohydrate calories. Eleven grams times four calories per gram equals 44 calories. Next multiply fat calories. Five grams times nine calories per gram equals 45 calories. Fat calories are 45 of the 120 calories. More that one-third of the calories are fat calories in 2% milk!

2. Check labels and avoid foods with more than three grams of fat per serving.
3. Buy 1% or skim milk.
4. Use oil-free salad dressings.
5. Change your cooking techniques to broiling, baking, steaming and microwaving to decrease your oil intake.
6. Remove skin from poultry since it is high in fat.
7. Use jellies or jams without butter on bread and avoid the fat

calories of butter and margarine.

8. Substitute low-fat or non-fat yogurt in place of ice cream for snacks.

9. Pretzels as a snack are very low in fat while potato chips have 10 times more fat.

10. In the cookie department, try graham crackers, fig bars and ginger snaps since these are low in fat.

< 5 >

How Do You Judge The Seriousness
Of A Back Attack?

Read about the rule of thumb that tells you
when you should try a home remedy to relieve pain.

How do you know how serious the injury is that generates a sudden attack of back pain? When should you see a doctor and when should you try a home remedy to relieve the pain?

There is a rule of thumb to follow and there are some symptoms that flash a warning light that your injury may be debilitating.

As I indicated in Chapter 2, most simple back pain will start to improve with a day or two of rest and some aspirin or Advil. If you discover the pain stays on and that you're taking more and more pills to relieve it, or if the pain is getting worse, call your physician.

Among the chief signals of back injury that flash a warning light are the foot drop and loss of bowel or bladder control. If you've injured your back and find that you drag your foot when you walk because your leg muscles cannot raise your toes, call your doctor immediately. Such a symptom is a sign of a serious neurological problem such as nerve impingement or a ruptured disc. Another danger signal is loss of bowel or bladder control. A person with any of these symptoms should go immediately to a spine doctor or a hospital emergency room. Ignoring signals like these could mean the permanent loss of muscular control over the affected parts of the body.

Pain that radiates down an arm or leg signifies a pinched nerve—perhaps from a bulging or ruptured disc. A ruptured disc doesn't necessarily require surgery to repair it. Most of the patients I see with ruptured discs recover from their back pain without surgery.

I mentioned earlier that prolonged bed rest adds to a back injury by producing inactivity that weakens muscles. For years, bed rest has been a common treatment for back injury. Even now, many doctors will advise a patient who has injured his back to take it easy. But extended bed rest is actually more harmful that it is helpful. In fact, studies on acute back pain show that two days of bed rest is as good as a week or more of reclining so that sprained muscles may relax and mend.

When bed rest and anti-inflammatories don't help you within a day or so, however, you should seek out a back specialist, because this is often a sign that something more serious is wrong. And never forget to heed the warning signs of serious trouble which I described.

To get the most out of only two days of bed rest, you need to take weight and pressure off the spine. Don't lie face down, for example, because this position still places some strain on your back. The position that best removes all body weight is to arrange yourself on your back with a pillow under your knees. The second best position is on your side with a pillow between your knees.

Occupy your mind with distracting ideas—pastimes that take your attention off your pain—watch TV, listen to music, read a thriller.

The initial treatment of your pain should be done by following an important rule: apply ice first, then heat. Ice is always applied during the first

48 hours because it slows swelling and inflammation that occurs after injury. It also acts as an anesthetic by numbing sore tissues. After 48 hours, however, ice loses some of its effectiveness. Heat is used after the first two days because it aids the healing process by increasing circulation and relaxing muscle spasms.

The Texas Back Institute has reported a great first aid tip with ice: Take several paper cups and fill them almost to the top with water. Put them in your freezer. When they are frozen, peel the edge of the cup back one inch, then gently apply the ice cup to the skin over the area of soreness on the back. Lie on your stomach with a pillow under your hips or lie on your side and have the person whose performing the service apply the ice in a circular motion over a six-inch area where you feel the pain. Avoid the area directly over the spine. Massage the area with the ice for about five minutes at a time.

The cold from the ice will make the veins in the tissue contract, reducing circulation. However, once the ice is removed the veins under the skin overcompensate and dilate, allowing blood to rush into the sore area. This blood, along with the oxygen it carries, will begin healing the damaged tissue.

As you have already concluded, I'm sure, this whole book is devoted to convincing the reader that exercise is the most beneficial remedy for back pain, and it is the best method to avoid weakness in the back that will make it more susceptible to injury. Numerous studies prove that exercise is more effective at treating simple back pain than passive methods such as rest and drugs. There are several reasons. One of them is that exercise restricts the source of pain to a smaller area. Exercise is the best way to concentrate the pain in a localized area, from a broad area, accelerate the healing process, prevent the injury from happening again, and reducing the severity of the pain.

Another important reason for exercise is that it stimulates the production of the body's own natural pain killers, called endorphins and encephalins. The presence of endorphins and other mood enhancers in the bloodstream falls off dramatically without exercise. To have your back in continuing good shape, you must make exercise part of a daily routine for both the painkilling benefits as well as for maintaining your strength and endurance.

In the following pages, you'll discover people who developed back injuries and what courses of action they followed to restore themselves to activity. These anecdotes help to demonstrate the regenerative powers of the back.

Also, you'll learn a little about the painful sciatica attack.

"But I Don't Have Any Back Trouble."

All too often I treat patients without any back problems but with back pain. Forced inactivity from another medical or personal problem has caused loss of spine strength and flexibility resulting in new-found back pain.

Take the case of Elizabeth. She is single and a minister at a large parish. Elizabeth prevents "burn out" by spending her time off paddling the lakes around Seattle in her canoe. Rock-hard and suntanned, she appears in robust health.

Abdominal pain one evening changed her life. Eight hours of cramping and pain brought her to the hospital where a diagnosis of appendicitis was made. A routine surgery was performed but her appendix had ruptured and peritonitis, a severe infection of the lining of the abdomen, set in.

Elizabeth remained in the hospital for two weeks on intravenous antibiotics. She had drains and tubes in more places than she cared to count. Her healthy body had been dealt a blow, but she recovered and felt her energy returning. Six weeks later she was ready for the water but sitting in the kayak caused back pain. Loading the light Kevlar kayak on her car was excruciating. She was referred to us for treatment by a friend.

Examination disclosed that Elizabeth's flexibility was 60 percent of normal and her aerobic endurance was near normal as a result of her water-sports and her bicycling. Unfortunately, her spine strength was only 50 percent of normal. With a strong upper body and a weak back, extra strain is placed on the "weak link" of the low back. Elizabeth was prescribed *Superwoman* exercises and extension exercises as seen on pages 84 and 85.

It took two months to restore the strength to her back and during the process, Elizabeth sanded and applied a gelcoat to a kayak she was building in her basement.

With her new-found back strength Elizabeth headed off into the San Juan Islands with her kayak for a long weekend. The only sounds she heard were the dip and drip of the paddle as she skimmed toward the distant islands.

Forced rest from any cause increases loss of muscle strength in the spine and other areas of the body. When her back muscles became weak, Elizabeth's vertebrae moved independently and often erratically rather than working as a unit. The result was instability of the back and back pain.

To treat the problem, Elizabeth's muscle tone needed to be restored and flexibility returned to normal. Because these two functions can be measured, Elizabeth was able to tell how much exercise she needed and how much was enough.

"A Pot Belly Makes A Good Stove."

"I'll take these penny loafers," Chris said.

The cordovan shell of the supple leather felt soft to his examining fingers. "Do you have one of those long-handled shoe horns?" he asked the clerk in the shoe department.

Chris experienced back pain whenever he tried to bend over to tie his shoes or pick up items from the floor. He squirmed around in his chair at work, first leaning on one arm rest then the other, then turning slightly side to side to find a comfortable position.

Fingering the shoes, he realized they did not fit his image as a successful banker. Although he had money, he had been worried about his health since he read about obesity.

Chris had taken the POT BELLY test in a throw-away magazine about executives and their life styles. The questions he pondered were, "How much was his oversized abdomen hurting him and would sit-ups make the pot belly go away?" "Besides preventing him from participating in sports, were there more problems with obesity?" He knew about the low back pain but assumed that was from getting older. He was pushing 40. He sipped and snacked during his evening in front of the TV while he read the *Wall Street Journal.*

The clerk returned with the long-handled shoe horn. Chris was impressed with himself for thinking to purchase an item that would allow him to get his shoes on easily. He hadn't been able to bend over and tie the laces for two years. At first his wife tied his shoes but Chris could sense her disappointment and frustration with him for not taking care of himself.

Then he turned in his wing-tips for loafers and although the loafers were not dressy, he could put them on without assistance.

Arriving home, Chris saw the yardstick in the closet when he hung up his suit coat. It reminded him of the pot belly test he had read in a magazine:

"While on your back on the floor, place a yardstick with one end on your breast bone and the other end on your knees. If you can't make both ends lie flat," the article advised, "then you have a pot belly."

"Okay," he admitted, "I have a pot belly. I can get rid of this," he resolved, "by doing sit-ups." He did six sit-ups then lay gasping on the floor. His out-of-shape muscles and added weight made the sit-ups nearly impossible and they hurt his back.

Chris rummaged through the waste basket for the magazine article. He found it and read: "The fat on your abdomen doesn't belong to your abdomen, it belongs to your mouth. To get rid of fat, you must change your eating habits as well as exercising."

Chris came to me and asked for help. I referred him to a bariatric physician, a doctor specializing in weight loss. To be successful with permanent weight loss many people such as Chris need a structured, supervised program. The weekly reinforcement and counseling help them understand why they are overweight, how the obesity keeps them in bondage and what can be done. Chris managed the life-style changes. He no longer ate while reading or watching TV. He picked healthier snacks and once again he was able to tie his shoes. Even vacuuming and picking up items from the floor did not cause pain.

In addition to his weight loss, we started Chris on a program of flexibility. His two greatest problems were back weakness because of excessive weight and inability to bend forward because of stiffness from the old pot belly. Losing the weight resulted in normal spine strength based on body weight (see Chapter 2). We taught him flexibility stretches for flexion (See pages 35 and 37). Chris followed his exercise prescription and became a participant in life rather than an observer. He swapped his favorite lounge chair for a bicycle seat and was exhilarated by his new life-style. He felt the wind in his face and heard the sounds of the rustling leaves in the overhead branches. He had forgotten these experiences of years past. "Maybe I'll try the Seattle to Portland bicycle ride next year," he thought.

Previous Spine Surgery With A Fusion. "If It Is Supposed To Help, Why Does It Keep Hurting?"

Leon's vision began to distort behind his fire-resistant face mask. His eyes were undamaged but perspiration was running down his face from the intense heat in building #4 of the chemical plant. His respirator clicked and vented as he breathed compressed air in his fire-proof suit.

He heard the cracking sound, looked up, then bent forward as the wooden ceiling collapsed striking him squarely across the shoulders. As the roof fell, the raging flames surged skyward in search of more oxygen.

Leon's partner saw him go down and pulled him to safety.

This was Leon's third injury as a firefighter. His back had exploded with pain. "Next time," he had been advised by his doctor, "you'll be having a fusion of your low back."

Because of the recurrent disc herniations in his spine and the loss of low back stability, a fusion operation was prescribed for Leon. Two metal plates were used to stop the abnormal low back motion. See the pictures on page 70. Despite the previous four laminectomies which had been performed on Leon's back, removing much of the bony supporting structure for the spine, the fusion did its job. It stopped the motion between the three lowest vertebrae in Leon's back. After the surgery he felt stiff. He was stiff! He wore a back brace while the fusion healed and then his doctor referred him for rehabilitation. After spine fusion, the back moves less in every direction. To increase the motion to normal would mean making the remaining vertebrae

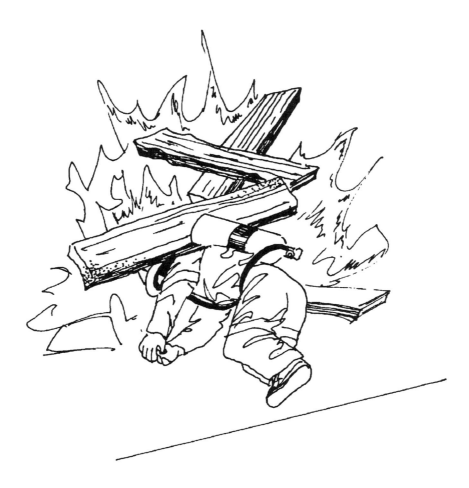

and discs perform more movement and work than they were designed to perform. As an example, the spine loses 40 percent of its motion if just two of the five discs and vertebrae are fused together.

Leon still had back pain but his severe leg pain was resolving. After successfully completing rehabilitation, he had a physical capacity test performed to see what kind of work he could do. He was disappointed to discover that his flexibility was only 60 percent of normal even though he had normal strength. He was advised to change to a less physically demanding

Leon Before Back Fusion

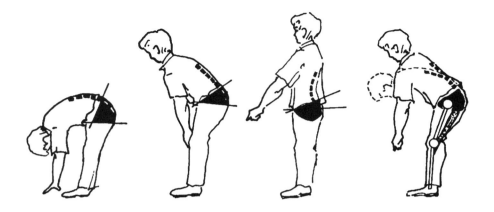

Illustration 52

Leon After Back Fusion

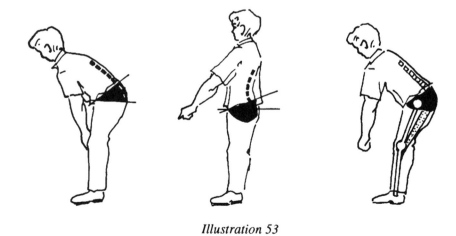

Illustration 53

job.

Returning to his doctor, he inquired, "Dr. Smith, why does my back keep hurting even though my legs feel so much better?"

"Spine surgery," Dr. Smith said, "with fusion is used to stop the nerves to the legs from being pinched where they start in the low back. The reason for the back pain is five-fold. First, when a fusion is performed, the fascia (pronounced "fash-uh") or shrink-wrap around the muscles is cut and may not return to its pre-surgery state. Secondly, muscles must be cut away from the bone in order to put metal plates or bone strips in place for the fusion. Thirdly, the low back loses one-fifth of its motion for each disc level fused. Fourth, sometimes the bone strips from the fusion or the screws holding the metal plates touch against a nerve. Lastly, the muscles running over the low back vertebrae are no longer stretched totally since much of the bony movement is lost. It is a feeling like only being able to do two-thirds of a yawn."

Leon's doctor again advised him to take a less physically-demanding job. The firefighter could have taken total disability but he chose instead to take a light-duty position as an instructor in *Basic Life Support* or C.P.R. This way he could remain around the "family" of smoke eaters he had come to love and not have to worry since he couldn't give one hundred percent to fighting fires.

Leon wanted to know what else he could do to help control his back pain. During a follow-up visit with the physician at the rehabilitation center, he was given several suggestions.

"Use your HGB," said the doctor.

"What?" questioned Leon.

The doctor continued. "We want you to focus on the HGB, the *Hamstring-Gluteal-Back* complex. These are the muscles on the back of the thigh, the back of the buttocks and the low back muscles. An easy way to strengthen these muscles is to put your car seat in an upright position. Slowly push back against the non-moving seat for eight seconds than relax. Move the seat back one notch farther and repeat. Do this in four or five positions. Don't drive while performing this exercise."

The doctor advised Leon that he would notice an increase in strength

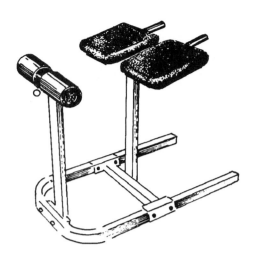

Illustration 54

in a few weeks, a decrease in his pain as the HGB muscles took over the work of the affected spine.

If you want to strengthen your low back muscles and use the Roman chair, illustration 54, raise only to a position parallel with the floor.

If you have access to a back machine like a Cybex, or Nautilus, see if you can find one that has a range limiting device to allow you to perform limited motion or isometric strengthening like you can use with the car seat.

Also pay attention to the proper lifting techniques noted in Chapter 8.

Sciatica, The Cursed Visitor

Sciatica (sigh-attic-uh), a painful word. Most folks get a nagging backache at times but a few unfortunate ones will develop sciatica, the sharp, gnawing pain that burns like a hot poker in the buttock and down the back of the leg to the knee, or to the foot.

The sciatic nerve is the largest nerve in the body, approximately equal to your thumb in diameter. When the sciatic nerve acts up, your entire life will be affected. Pain control will be your only goal.

What causes pain in this long nerve? See illustration 55. This side view of the low back shows three nerves from the spinal cord to the legs. Five spinal nerves make up the sciatic nerve. Anything that pinches or inflames

Causes of Sciatic Pain

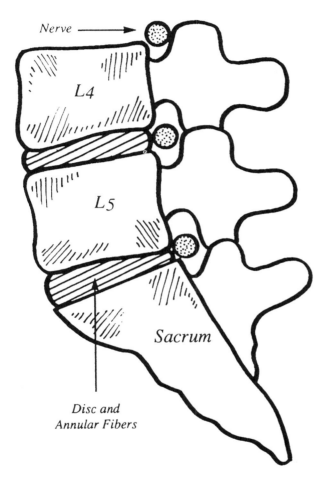

Nerve

L4

L5

Sacrum

*Disc and
Annular Fibers*

*Anything that pinches or
inflames the nerves from the
spinal cord may cause
sciatica.*
1. Bone spur.
*2. Inflammation from a
damaged disc.*
3. A "worn out" disc.
*4. A muscle strain with
bleeding or bruising around
the nerve.*
*5. Disc herniation or rupture
pushing out backward against
the nerve.*
*6. Weak back muscles that
allow abnormal motion of the
spine with pressure on these
nerves.*

Illustration 55

these nerves may cause sciatica such as a bone spur, inflammation from a damaged disc, a worn out or "degenerated disc," a herniated disc pushing out backward against the nerve or weak back muscles that permit abnormal motion of the vertebrae.

The herniated disc is what most doctors think of when you develop this agonizing pain. If you have sciatica, see your doctor. He or she will want to perform a thorough evaluation to find out why you hurt. If you have a herniated or ruptured disc, you still won't need surgery in 90 percent of the cases. Take heart, your doctor can find the cause of this problem most of the time and usually can treat you with a spine function restoration program that will involve strength, flexibility, aerobics and muscular endurance exercises. Even degenerating discs and muscle tears usually respond to this type of treatment. See chapters 9, 10, 11 and 12 for more information.

How A Disc Herniation Or Rupture Occurs

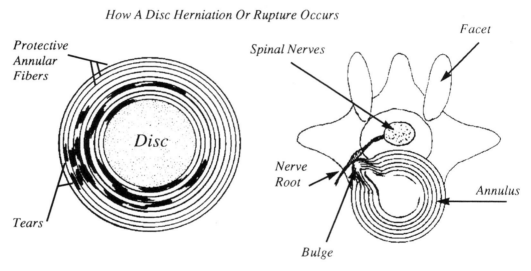

Illustration 56

Disc ruptures do not occur from one injury but rather are the straw that broke the camel's back. On the left above, there are several black areas of fiber tears, each from a small strain or injury. Over time a series of small tears may be compounded into a strain or injury that tears the fibers all the way to the outside of the protective annular fibers. When this happens the disc material is pushed out and it pushes on nerves in the spinal canal producing back pain and or leg pain.

Football: The Glory Days—Osteoarthritis

The "high" B. J. experienced during his professional football days was never duplicated in his work as a car salesman. People came from miles away to buy a car from him and talk sports. His days with the Seattle Seahawks were the greatest moments of his life. Never mind that he was never home and was constantly harassed for autographs in restaurants. He felt important.

Selling cars was okay, but his weekends were spent in front of the large screen TV at home or at work as he watched all the games. His life centered around football. He had played five years of pro ball, longer than average. During his career he had broken nine different bones on the playing field but they had healed and he continued in the body-bruising sport.

When B. J. opened his eyes every morning he knew he would have to put himself through the same painful routine of forcing his creaking body to move. The years of bone-jarring high school, college and professional football had taken their toll on his body. He was so stiff each day that he took a 30 minute shower with scorching hot water to try to loosen his muscles. It helped. He followed the shower with 20 minutes of stretching, then he could sit down for a cup of coffee and read the sports page.

He was paying the price for the thousands of times he had been tackled and thrown to the ground. Being a fullback was not all glory; most of it was hard work. B. J. had pain for days after every pro game. It was expected. If you weren't sore, you weren't putting out. His spine and discs degenerated as a result of trauma from the blocks and tackles he endured.

After retirement from football he had become inflexible and his muscles tightened up each time he lay down or sat for any period of time. He noticed that sliding into a cold car on the parking lot made his back sore. It was painful for him to bend or twist.

"I never hurt this much when I was playing football," he told his doctor. "What is the matter?"

His doctor did an exam including X-rays of his back which showed that B. J. had developed severe arthritis with spurs (bony growths) that pushed against some of the nerves in his back. He also had degenerating

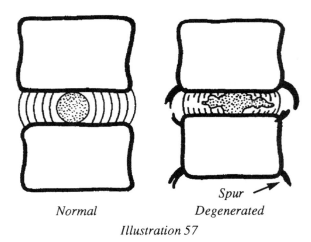

Side View Of Disc And Its Vertebrae

Normal   *Spur* →

Degenerated

Illustration 57

(wearing out) discs. See illustration 57. The arthritis could not be reversed, but there was hope.

"How much exercise do you get every day, B. J.?" asked his doctor.

"I do stretches every morning."

"No, I mean real exercise, like walking, biking, lifting weights, or swimming?"

"Well, I don't do any of those things anymore," B. J. said, a little sheepishly. He thought of the three hours of practice and exercise he had gone through daily for the 13 years he played football. Now he considered himself fortunate if he didn't have to walk more than 50 feet to go into a store. "I really haven't done anything," he said.

His doctor nodded. "I rarely see anyone in my office for back pain as long as they are in school. Once they graduate and begin jobs, they begin to have back problems because of inactivity. Inactive muscles become shortened and tight and cause pain. You also have arthritis from all the years of football. I want you to see a sports medicine physician to find out what you can do to get relief from some of the pain."

The sports medicine expert to whom B. J. was referred placed him immediately on a strengthening program to restore his back to normal function. An examination revealed that B. J. had only 40 percent of normal back strength and he was not doing all of the correct stretches. His new program included trunk strengthening three times a week and stretching twice daily, first in the morning and then before bed. In a week, B. J. breathed easier with significantly less pain. His mobility increased and he started to feel good again.

B. J.'s stretches for low and mid-back flexibility were performed on a low back strengthening machine, a Cybex. He was amazed and glad to discover that deterioration in muscles could be reversed through exercise. Now, his strength is back to normal and he plays some weekend football again. He uses a VCR and records all the games while he is out exercising and he gets his "high" from coaching Little Guy Football and running with the boys. He's a hero and they benefit from his years of experience.

Frequent injuries to his back caused damage to the small facet (fuh-set) joints. The little joints developed arthritis from repeated damage and became painfully inflamed. As the inflammation persisted, it spread to higher and lower areas in B. J.'s back. See illustration 58.

Your body is constantly trying to heal itself. When you injure the facet joints, they become moveable and roughened. When a joint moves beyond its normal boundary, the capsule around it is stretched and torn. Your back works at stabilizing itself by growing bony spurs from one vertebrae to another. When the spurs from one vertebra meet with another vertebra, you become stiff because the vertebra have less motion between them. This is called the stabilization process and often your pain will decrease when you become stabilized. Usually this happens when you are in your sixties or seventies.

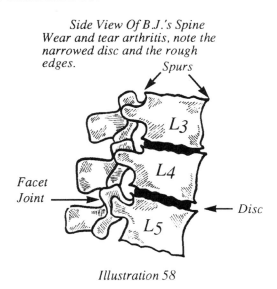

Side View Of B.J.'s Spine
Wear and tear arthritis, note the narrowed disc and the rough edges.

Spurs

L3

L4

Facet Joint

Disc

L5

Illustration 58

During the years before stabilization, you can control the pain with strengthening and stretching.

Why do so many doctors recommend rest for injuries to the back? Initially, medical studies showed that there was less pressure on the discs of the low back when a patient was lying down. Based on that information, physicians have recommended bed rest up to two weeks for low back pain. It is now known that the more time spent in bed, the slower the recovery. Twenty years ago, patients spent three to five times as much time in hospitals as they do now. Healing rates are quicker now and there are less complications with short hospital stays. The same is true for low back pain. If your low back pain is not relieved after a day or two of rest, you need to take a new approach to resolving the problem.

Since only one or two percent of back problems are severe disc ruptures, the remaining 98 percent of people should keep moving. By continuing activity, you will promote better circulation and blood flow to the injured area as well as maintain your muscle strength and flexibility. Follow the suggestions for increasing low back flexibility, strength and endurance. Measure your progress frequently. You will soon find yourself back in motion.

Real people, real problems, real solutions. With the current information regarding measurement of spine function, you can determine your own areas of weakness and then strengthen them with a specific program. As the function of your back approaches normal, your pain will decrease and your capabilities will increase. You will find yourself back in action.

< 6 >

The "Bad" Reputation Of Herniated
Or Ruptured Discs

*It's not true that ruptures always
prevent people from sports or heavy work.*

The person who has suffered a herniated disc is apt to regard advice about functional restoration of the back through exercise as inapplicable to him. Yet millions of people play in professional sports and work in heavy labor with ruptured or herniated discs.

How can this be? You'll find the answer in the following explanation of how discs work and in the anecdotes about people who suffered disc injuries and recovered to continue the activities they pursued before they were hurt.

As you know, the spine is composed of 24 bones called vertebrae and the sacrum. Picture these bones, like blocks, piled in a column on top of one another. Without shock absorbers, these bones would eventually fracture and break from the downward force of striking together when you jar them as you walk, jump or run. That's why there are shock absorbers situated between the vertebrae, called discs.

The discs can take a lot of hammering without serious injury. But without knowing it you can harm your back through actions that repeatedly squash the discs causing the inner spongy material to break through the outer rings. Even then, you may be unaware of the injury and continue the bad habits of poor posture, improper lifting methods and lack of invigorating exercise until a bulge suddenly occurs in the pushed-out disc material and puts pressure on a nearby nerve connected to the spinal cord. When this happens, you'll know it because the sudden electric pain may grab you with an awful clutching spasm that will bend you over and take your breath away.

Herniation of the disc can occur when you put pressure on an already weakened or squashed disc by lifting something heavy without back muscles strong enough to take the load. You could be lifting a bag of groceries from the back of your car with weakened back muscles when it happens. More frequently, the herniation occurs as the result of some trauma. When the pulpy center of the disc is squeezed out of the disc wall and puts pressure on adjacent nerves, the sudden pain is excruciating. There is no experience that quite compares to it.

It is worth explaining that there is no such thing as a "slipped disc," a phrase often used to describe a herniated disc. The description implies that a disc has slipped out of place and can be restored to its proper position by a doctor who knows exactly what to do. The fact is, discs can't slip because they are attached to the vertebrae above and below with strong connective tissue.

It is important for everyone to know that once a disc is torn, it cannot repair itself. Normally, a disc is self-lubricating and injury resistant—it can take a lot of shock—but while the pain of injury can be relieved, the serious damage done to a disc can be permanent. That is why flexibility and aerobic exercise are so important. The circulating blood and the vigorous action of moving muscles help the disc to lubricate itself and they keep healthy from the increased blood flow to the the areas surrounding the disc space.

This remains true even as you grow older. Actually, blood stops flowing to the disc about age 20. As a result, the disc can dry out, become flatter, more brittle and more susceptible to injury. Blood circulating around the disc from exercise keeps the disc as healthy as possible.

Despite the fact that serious damage to a disc can be permanent, the fact is most disc injuries and problems can be treated without surgery! In the following vignettes and simplified diagrams, you'll see how herniated discs occur and what really happens to the back. Armed with this information, you'll understand more about your own back and you'll see that you don't have to abandon an active life. Discs don't stay young forever, but you can do a lot to protect them.

Triathletes Have Staying Power

Karen looked forward to the week at Elderhostel, an educational program including room and board. It provided the opportunity to study the Columbia ice field near Jasper and Lake Louise in Alberta, Canada. An optional leg of her trip involved a 10-mile bike ride up Mt. Edith Cavell near Jasper using low-geared mountain bicycles.

Karen was in great shape. She was involved with the Master's Triathalon series of bicycling, running and swimming. She and a few others had accepted the challenge of the mountain. The ride up was difficult but the mountain meadows with their blankets of wild flowers were a marvelous reward.

Coming down the mountain was exciting with the hair-pin turns and switchbacks. During hard braking for a switchback, Karen's front caliper brake pad overheated, melted and popped out of its holder. She had lost almost 70 percent of her stopping power and was only able to slow slightly before the switchback. Unable to maneuver the sharp left turn, she shot over the edge of the mountain road.

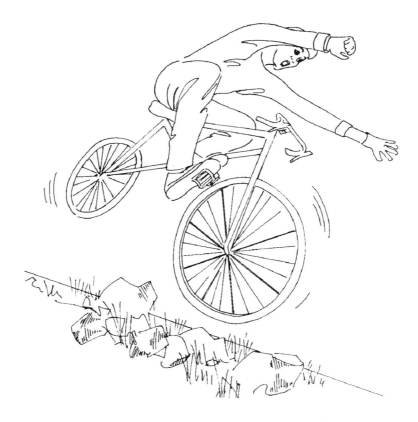

"Oh no!" she thought, "I think I'm dead." She couldn't remember what happened next but passers-by who saw her fly through the air say she landed 40 feet below on the shoulder of the road while still sitting on the bicycle.

The wheels collapsed, the frame shattered and Karen was thrown to the pavement. Her bicycle helmet protected her head but she suffered a fractured arm and foot and ruptured three discs in her lower back.

Two days later her mind lifted out of the fog as the swelling subsided around her brain. Disoriented, she tried to get up but was unable. Taking her bearings, she found herself in a hospital bed with casts on her arm and leg. Her back throbbed with each beat of her heart.

Studies performed while she was unconscious showed three mid-line disc herniations with extension or pushing off to the right with loss of right leg reflexes. See illustration 60. Her doctor advised her that surgery was not indicated for the discs but it would take several months for the pain to subside.

Injured discs give off inflammatory chemicals that produce swelling and pain. Several months often elapse between the time these chemicals are produced and the time that the discs "burn themselves out."

Karen was advised to start on an exercise program. Ten weeks elapsed before her leg fracture healed. In the meantime, she walked with a cane and a walking cast while she waited for the bones to mend. Karen knew what the phrase, "cabin fever" meant. She anticipated getting out of the house, back into her sports and onto her bicycle. She knew she would lose her nerve for bicycling if she didn't return to the saddle soon.

Her bones healed as the rains came to western Oregon. Then, she began with short neighborhood rides. For her longer excursions, she wore a wetsuit with a Gore-Tex shell to keep her bones warm during the two and three hour intervals she was exposed to pounding rains.

The following July, Karen attacked the Timberline Highway, a six-mile twisting roadway from Government Camp, Oregon to Timberline Lodge.

Anatomy Of Karen's Back Injury

The nerve root openings are made smaller by the discs that rupture producing pain and loss of reflexes. This usually improves over time without surgery.

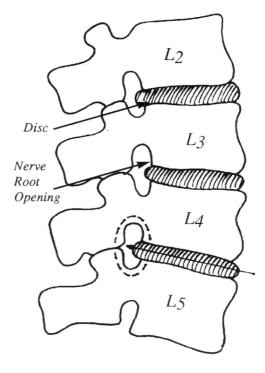

Illustration 60

climb through the cloud cover out of the rain into the bright sunshine. Never had she appreciated Timberline Lodge more than that day with its backdrop against snow-packed Mt. Hood.

Karen's new bicycle had high-quality brakes but she was still squeamish about the ride down the mountain. She took it slow and was grateful to reach Government Camp where she stopped for lunch.

While lunching she remembered what it had taken in devotion to exercise to bring herself back to bicycling fitness. She had performed extension exercises twice daily. See illustrations 61 through 65. She had bicycled to increase back strength and she had walked for one hour daily as soon as her casts were removed.

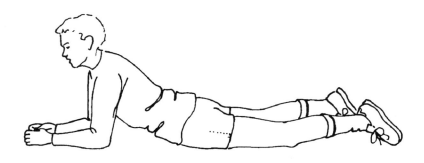

Illustrations 61 and 62

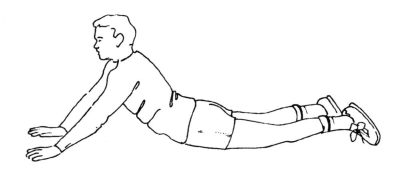

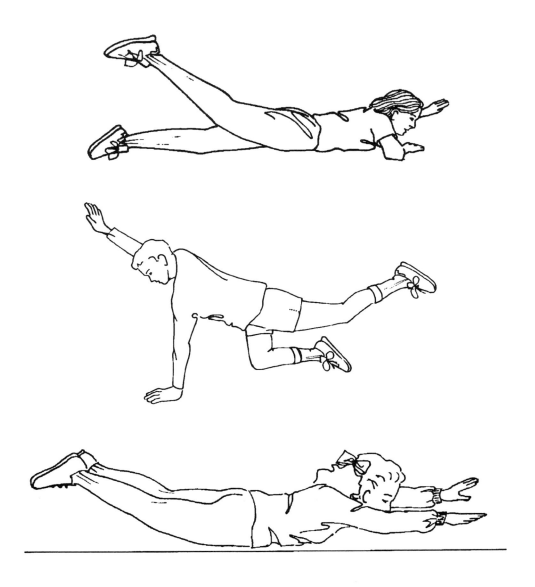

Illustrations 63, 64 and 65

She had been advised to purchase a rowing machine to help build back strength and she used it daily while she listened to the news. She started rowing gradually and increased slowly as she could tolerate the physical stress. When she reached 15 minutes per day, her back pain abated. Then she decided that her back was worth one hour daily in effort and exercise because it gave her 23 painless hours in return.

When the doctors examined her after the accident they discovered that the ruptured or herniated discs in Karen's back pinched the nerves to the right leg slightly but did not cause any weakness in the leg. As a result no surgery was performed. Her reflexes returned to normal and although she had back pain when she awakened each morning, she was determined to keep moving and enjoy her athletics. Several months after her mountain accident she opened an envelope she found in her mailbox. It was a flyer that showed pictures of the desert in bloom. Elderhostel was going to Death Valley to study the desert flora and fauna.

"I'd better buy some thorn-proof bicycle tubes to prevent flat tires," she thought.

The W.P.G.A. - A Perfect Place To Get Strokes

Nancy had her head down as she addressed the ball. Only the sound of the wind dancing in the trees was heard. More than one thousand bystanders were hushed as she started her backswing. She had bogeyed the previous hole and did not have a chance at first place money unless she could birdie the hole in front of her.

The lush fairway stretched out with its rolling hills while sand traps protected most of the green. To complicate the situation, the fairway dog-legged slightly to the left at 150 yards. Nancy had noticed the flag above the clubhouse minutes before. It was unfurled and held straight by the wind. That meant, Nancy knew, that the wind was at least 13 miles per hour. It was coming from her left up the dogleg. She would have to compensate for the wind and the dogleg and risk everything to birdie the hole.

She kept her focus on the ball while using her powers of mental imaging to see the ball soar straight down the fairway to the dogleg where it would turn left. Rather than let her near-perfect form drive the ball, she chose to put more force into the drive by violently contracting her trunk muscles to get an extra 50 or 75 yards.

It was working. She felt it when the face of the driver made contact with the ball. The ever so slight left spin on the ball made it turn gently left at the dogleg. "If the wind would only hold up for a few seconds," she hoped. There was a momentary lull in the breeze as the ball made a final effort to reach the green. Five feet from the green it stopped and rested. The rush of adrenaline from the near-perfect drive prevented her from feeling the burning in her low back.

Her heart was pounding. She still had a chance. She had perfect position. Could she chip her ball into the hole she wondered? A chip shot could keep her in this tournament. Myrtle Beach was her favorite course. When she struck it, the ball pitched upward and landed as softly as a butterfly with sore feet. It was only eight inches from the cup as it rolled slowly to the edge of the hole and teetered before dropping out of sight.

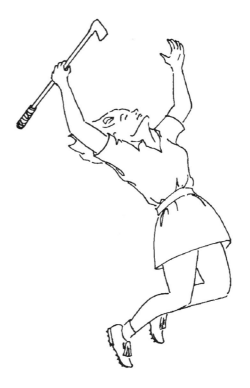

Nancy leaped into the air with excitement. When she landed she felt the penetrating pain in her low back as the third lumbar disc herniated. She broke out in a cold sweat in spite of the 80 degree morning. Using her years of discipline and focus, she forced herself to ignore the pain and continue with the tournament. When the first round was finished, she skipped the 19th hole and the reporters and headed to the club house to get a massage. The massage helped stop the muscle spasm and she scheduled another one for later that evening and early in the morning one hour before tee time.

Nancy's Injury

Sideview of the low back showing the ruptured disk pushing backward on the nerves. This injury often occurs after a strenuous twisting motion.

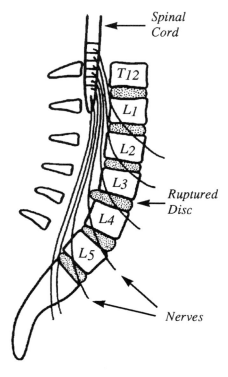

Spinal Cord

T12

L1

L2

L3

Ruptured Disc

L4

L5

Nerves

Illustration 67

She picked up some ibuprofen, an anti-inflammatory medication, and took two immediately. They did not help much. She called her physician and was told to take four every six hours. Four tablets helped some and she used the ice packs on her low back between massages. Her physician suggested she see a local doctor who treated the professional golfers when they were in town.

After a thorough exam, she was advised she had some loss of sensation in her legs due to a pinched nerve or a ruptured disc but at this time there was no reason to think she would need surgery. She was given a prescription for low dose prednisone, a potent anti-inflammatory agent. The prednisone helped her finish the tournament.

She came in third place. The money helped pay her expenses for the tournament she had just finished and for the next. She knew that everyone outside of professional golf thought that winning $200,000 per year would allow a person to live like a queen. The fact was that her expenses used up 60 percent of the money. The constant travel, entertainment and the lifestyle prevented her from being wealthy even with a large income.

When Nancy returned home she went to her private physician, Diane Feinstein. Diane performed a physical exam with special focus on Nancy's back and ordered an MRI scan to document the small disc herniation. It was a midline disc herniation but was not causing any significant neurologic damage. See illustration 67. Diane started Nancy on an aerobic exercise program on a Nordic Track machine to improve the blood supply to the spine during healing and to keep her muscles in tone for her tournaments.

"And Nancy, if you have any weakness in your legs or your foot seems to scrape the floor when you walk, get in to see me immediately. That might mean you are having more problems with the disc in your low back," said Diane.

Nancy continues to use the Nordic Track to keep her back in shape and the blood flowing in the space surrounding the damaged disc.

Powerlifting Was His Game

Arnold was a powerlifter. He had lifted 560 pounds from the floor using opposing hand grips on the bar after cinching up his six-inch-wide leather weight-lifting belt. Because his name was Arnold and since he spent two hours daily working with weights, he was constantly teased that he didn't look like Arnold Schwartzenegger, the body-building champion. He didn't mind. In fact, he seemed to enjoy the extra attention.

Arnold had a second hobby. He enjoyed tinkering with old cars. It filled his evening and kept his maintenance costs minimal. Arnold had been working on the transmission of his old car. He had taken it off the blocks and was washing it in the driveway. His two-year-old son was playing in the water behind the car. The driveway was on an incline and as Arnold scrubbed road tar off the passenger door, he heard a loud metal snap and the car started to roll backward. He ran behind the car and lifted it up by the bumper while

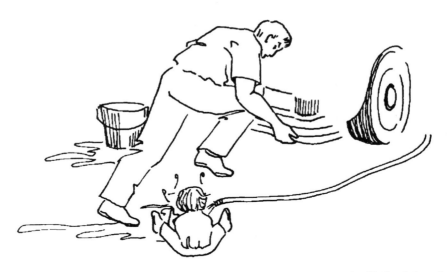

leaning his weight into the vehicle to stop it. His son, unmindful of the danger his father had prevented, continued to splash in the water. Arnold felt two pops in his low back as he pushed with all his strength to protect his son from the rolling vehicle.

The car stopped. Arnold yelled for someone to help. A neighbor, seeing what had happened, rushed over and picked up the youngster. The neighbor then put blocks behind the wheels to halt the car on the incline.

Fiery low back pain developed in Arnold's back. He couldn't sit down and he couldn't tolerate standing. He had to lie first on one side, then the other keeping a pillow between his knees. Arnold self-tested the strength in his legs. He was familiar with exercise physiology and since his leg strength was unimpaired, he wasn't sure what had happened, but he was almost certain that he hadn't injured himself enough to need any surgery.

"Keep moving," was the powerlifting adage. Arnold kept moving after two days of rest. The stiffness decreased with stretching and deep massage but the pain persisted.

He decided to see a physician. After a thorough exam and imaging studies, Arnold was told he had three ruptured discs in his back but they had ruptured into the bone above each disc rather than backward into the area near the spinal cord. See illustration 70. He was advised that stretching and light

Side View Of The Back
Injured Area

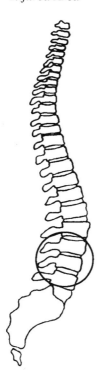

Illustration 69

exercise would speed the healing so he worked at pool therapy.

He walked for one hour daily in the local pool and participated in the pool running program to restore function to his back. While in the water he did not have pressure on his back from the weight of his body and was able to exercise nearly pain-free. He purchased an Aqua Vest to wear which helped keep him upright while

Anatomy Of Arnold's Injury
Disc is pushed up into the bone above.

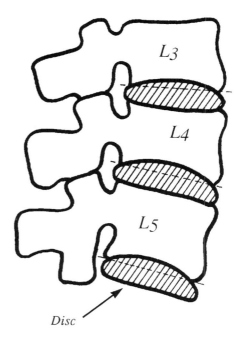

Illustration 70

performing the exercises. Arnold enjoyed the pool therapy so much he incorporated it into his powerlifting program.

Arnold keeps in excellent shape working on call as a stevedore unloading ships at the Port of Portland.

How do you know when you need surgery for a herniated disc? If you have incapacitating leg pain following a back injury or if weakness develops in either leg or foot, you may be a candidate for surgery. If one foot scrapes on the ground as you walk or seems to "catch" as you walk, then you may have a surgical problem. If either leg or foot feels "heavy" and does not work properly or if you are noticing a progressive change in one leg or foot, then see a doctor.

Most of the time a disc herniation does not mean having to give up the active life or being an invalid. Surgeons do not perform disc surgery as often as in the past. Ninety-six percent of back injuries do not need surgery. If you are not sure if your back needs surgery or rehabilitation, ask your doctor. No doctor has all the answers and will usually welcome a second opinion. If you are advised to have a back surgery, get a second opinion. If you are advised you need to participate in a "back program," then do it.

Remember, after three days of rest, each additional day of rest and inactivity results in the loss of three percent of your strength and flexibility and you have to work much harder to restore the lost function.

Instead, keep active with walking or pool therapy to stimulate your muscles and keep your heart in good shape for pumping nutrients to the healing tissues of the back.

< 7 >

Osteoporosis and Back Pain —
Fragile and Frail Bones

*A preventable disease that makes women susceptible
to hip and vertebrae fractures.*

The word osteoporosis conjures up the image of a little old lady, stooped forward and shuffling stiffly along with her cane. A cub scout den mother a few years ago, she enjoyed hiking with her family and watching her children participate in athletic events. What went wrong? How did she so quickly become round shouldered and bent? What could she have done to avoid the crippling effects of the disease that strikes women, bows their backs and makes fragile bones vulnerable to ordinary stresses? How can the average

This picture shows the change in the spine posture and curves that result from the fractures.

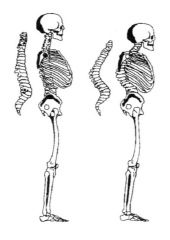

Normal   Fractures
Illustration 71

woman ward off osteoporosis, or reverse its devastating effects on the health of the spine?

What is osteoporosis? Who gets it? What can you do about it? *Osteo* means bone and *porosis* means porous. It describes

Normal Bone - Microscopic

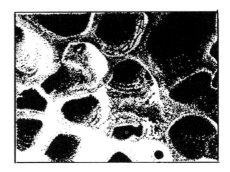

Illustration 72A

Bone With Osteoporosis - Microscopic
There is less bone mass.

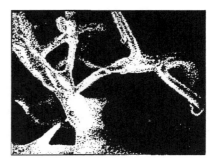

Illustration 72B

a condition — mostly in women— in which the bones become too porous or too fragile. Don't underestimate the cost of osteoporosis. Older women — and men also — can lose their independence, spend lots of their money and sometimes lose their lives. Osteoporosis is a symptom of a metabolic problem. It is the excessive loss of calcium from the bones that may result in pain or fractures or both. Back pain is a signal that something is wrong.

This signal does not mean you must give up a vigorous, active life. Osteoporosis is a loss of the bone minerals. The victim loses bone calcium faster than she can replace it. The woman who suffers from osteoporosis over time develops weakness in her bones and becomes susceptible to fracture.

One third of all women over 65 will have fractures of the vertebrae in their back as a result of osteoporosis. Fifteen percent will have hip fractures. That is the same number as all women who will have breast, uterine and ovarian cancer combined.

Men have only a five percent lifetime risk of osteoporosis because the male hormone testosterone keeps bones hard.

Conditions which predispose to rapid bone loss such as estrogen deficiency affect the spine bones first then the hip bones. Bone is made up of a protein frame like a house under construction with the 2 x 4 walls in place. Minerals of calcium then line up along this 2 x 4 protein frame to produce bone strength.

What makes your bones soft? Bone loss is a result of immobilization through illness, space travel or inadequate amounts of estrogen. The risk of Caucasian women sustaining a fracture from osteoporosis is one in three! The Black population has harder bones with infrequent fractures while the Oriental population falls between the Caucasian and Black populations.

If you are a female, white and thin, then you are at risk for osteoporosis. The highest risk group includes those women who:
>   1. Have had their ovaries removed.
>   2. Have family members and relatives with osteoporosis.
>   3. Have been taking some form of cortisone for a long period.
>   4. Have had hyperthyroidism (overactive thyroid).
>   5. Are inactive or sedentary.
>   6. Smoke or drink.

If you have osteoporosis, you want to avoid the second type of osteoporosis that frequently occurs, *osteoporosis of atrophy* caused by inactivity from resting because you have pain. If you have ever broken a bone and worn a cast, you may have noticed how quickly your leg or arm muscles became smaller. Because the muscle around the injured bone was resting, it

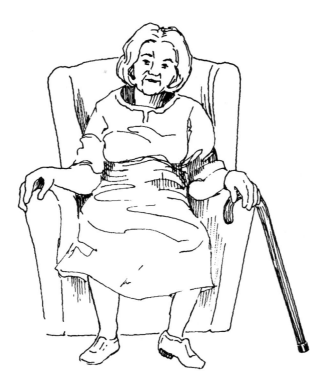

was not required to work and became lazy and weak. Bones develop their strength and hardness from being used. If you are not using the muscles that pull on the bones, then the bones will lose their strength and their calcium and become weak and thin.

Thousands of elderly women with osteoporosis spend their days in a recliner or on their favorite couch. They developed osteoporosis and then rested to allow healing of the vertebrae in their back. Because of this rest their spine muscles became weak. As a result, they experienced more pain, so they rested more. Osteoporosis from low estrogen, plus osteoporosis of atrophy cause a downward spiraling, vicious cycle. Weak bones attract injury; rest induces weaker bones.

The ideas in this chapter will help you deal with the frustration that prompts such complaints as "I hurt too much to pick up my grandchildren." "They don't understand!" "I can't lift a ladder anymore." " Everything feels heavier than it did five years ago." "What can I do?"

Exercise For Compression Fractures

Fifty-one-year-old Amy had low and middle back pain. She worked as a maid in a hotel and was making a bed when the pain started. She was bent over from the waist when she felt a "pop" in her back below her bra line, then burning pain radiated up and down her spine. Muscle spasms developed around the injured vertebra as the pain became intolerable.

Amy reported the injury and hobbled home. The next day she had increased pain and stiffness in her back. She called her doctor who took X-rays of her spine. They showed the compressed vertebra in her mid to low back. See illustration 74.

"What can I do to stop the pain?" she asked. Her physician advised her to take prescription analgesics. He said she had experienced a compression fracture that would hurt like any other fracture. The front of the vertebra bone was crushed into itself. It would heal, but it would take time. During

Spine, Normal And With Osteoporosis

Darker on X-ray means loss of calcium, L2, L3, L4 are compressed on top and bottom. L5 has been crushed so appears more white on X-ray as the crushing caused it to become more dense.

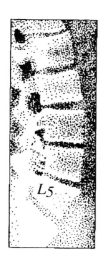 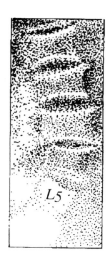

Illustration 74

the healing period, Amy was to follow prescribed exercises. She was not to lie around while she recuperated. Here is the prescription Amy's physician gave her:

• Make exercise part of your day. • Start gently and work up. • Make it fun, make it enjoyable. • Pick your best time of day.• Wear soft, comfortable shoes. • Set realistic goals. • Don't expect big results too soon. • Persevere, you can do it. • Reward yourself for your efforts.

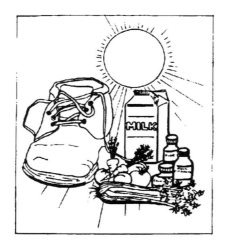

"How should I start?" Amy asked.

"Pick an activity that you enjoy and set realistic goals," her doctor told her. "As your fitness improves, you can add additional activities." Good exercises to start with Amy was advised, were bicycling and walking. She started with five blocks of walking daily and was to add one additional block every fourth day. If that was too painful, she was to begin on a stationary bicycle at 60-80 pedal revolutions per minute. Ride for three minutes the first day and add one minute every fourth day.

The important thing about the advice Amy's doctor gave her was his realization that exercise was the key to her recuperation. If you suffer from an osteoporosis related injury, exercise is your ticket to recovery. And just as you can hear the enthusiastic voices of children on a playground as they are exercising, you can make exercise fun. If the exercise is enjoyable, you are likely to follow through with it.

If you love water, then visit the pool. The beauty of the exercise prescription is that it can be adjusted to fit your preferences. If you are a night owl, then exercise in the evening when you feel your best. If you always greet the sunrise with a cheery smile, then exercise in the morning. Find an exercise buddy or a group who can share your enthusiasm for life and activity.

Don't expect too much too soon. It doesn't matter that you can't walk two miles after two weeks. The important thing is that you keep trying. At first, exercise makes stale muscles sore so you may feel worse before you begin to feel better.

Warm up before exercising. Remember your muscles are like a garden hose. A warm hose is supple and flexible while a cold hose is stiff and brittle and is more easily damaged. Walk in place in the house for a few minutes to get the blood moving before walking outside on a cold day.

Reinforce your success by rewarding yourself frequently. Treat yourself to small rewards such as a new magazine or a low-fat snack. Consider a few minutes in the hot tub or get a massage to relax your tired muscles. It will revive you.

Which exercise is best? For you, the best exercise is the one you will do and will continue to enjoy. First, restore your injured area to near-normal function. Then add another exercise such as low-impact aerobics. Consider a day-long bicycle tour with frequent stops to enjoy the scenery and the country stores.

If you wish to prevent osteoporosis, follow the strengthening program in Chapter 9. If you have osteoporosis now, then use the exercises in Chapter 3 which are designed more for toning. If you have a fracture, you want to prevent additional fractures from strenuous exercises. Use the toning exercises in Chapter 3.

How much exercise does it take? The greatest gains come from beginning any exercise. Being a top athlete is not important when recovering from injury. More importantly, moderate exercise will increase the blood flow to injured tissues and speed healing.

Amy's doctor placed her on a sound exercise program to speed healing and add interest during her recovery period. She walked, bicycled and used Thera-bands. Exercises like running and jumping rope when you have a compression fracture are inappropriate. Heavy weight lifting is not recommended. Low-impact activities restore blood flow and speed recovery.

Amy returned to work two months after her injury. She took 2,000 milligrams of calcium and walked daily to maintain a good blood supply and positive balance of calcium.

"I should have known better than to let this happen," Kathy thought as she lay on the stretcher looking up at the bright emergency room lights.

Kathy was a surgical nurse. She had had a total hysterectomy including removal of her ovaries twelve years before for uncontrolled uterine bleeding. At first, she had taken the prescribed estrogen pills but as they did not make her feel any better, she had stopped taking them when her prescription expired.

She had been lifting a heavy cardiac surgery tray out of the sterilizer when she felt the jolt in her back that took away her breath. She dropped the sterilized tray of metal instruments to the floor with a loud crash that brought operating room personnel to her side. She dropped to the floor on her hands and knees trying to take pressure off the compressed vertebra in her back. Even a deep breath caused pain.

Transported to the emergency room on a stretcher, Kathy was X-rayed and the film showed a compression fracture of T12 or thoracic vertebra number 12. See

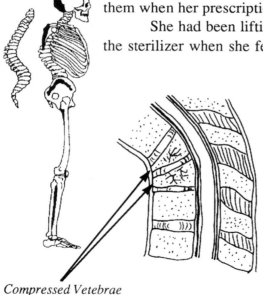

Compressed Vetebrae

Illustrations 77A and 77B

illustrations 77A and 77B. If the front of a few vertebrae crush with compression fractures, the resulting injury to the spine can develop a stooped-forward posture in the victim. A 24-hour urine test for calcium showed Kathy was losing calcium faster than she was ingesting it—a sure sign that her injury was serious.

In consultation with her doctors, Kathy learned that she would have to take responsibility for healing her back, avoiding another fracture and choosing to follow a diet that would replace calcium in her body. Kathy wanted to avoid another fracture so she exercised with a Thera-band until she could walk. See illustrations 78A and 78B. She supplemented her diet with calcium-rich foods and calcium supplements. Foods loaded with calcium include milk and dairy products, fish and shellfish, such as oysters, sardines, and shrimp. Dark green vegetables such as turnip greens, mustard greens, kale, broccoli and collards contain high amounts of calcium.

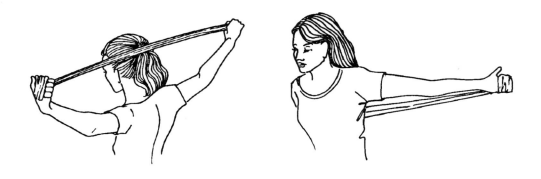

Illustrations 78A and 78B

She started taking estrogen and a flouride supplement to harden the bones. Though she knew the flouride was controversial, Kathy was anxious to do everything possible to prevent a new fracture as a result of weakened bones.

A medication called Didronel, marketed by Norwich-Eaton was

prescribed for Kathy. Didronel is more effective than estrogen and is supplemented with calcium. Ask your doctor about Didronel or Etidronate, the generic name. Etidronate *increases* bone mass while estrogen only *prevents* loss of bone mass.

Kathy loved swimming but couldn't get into the freestyle position because of the pain. Instead, she moved around the pool slowly and each day spent more time trying to swim on her back. This position took pressure off the injured vertebra. By consciously taking control of her future, Kathy had made the decision to prevent a hip fracture from osteoporosis, a common occurrence in older women. She was taking responsibility for her good health.

With new priorities in her life, Kathy returned to work after six weeks. She had to take care of herself first, she realized, before she could take care of others. She kept her estrogen, calcium and flouride by her toothbrush so she would remember to take them. She exercised daily after work. If she worked on call during the night in surgery, she'd take a nap the following afternoon then would exercise. At the fitness center, she could enjoy the company of others committed to the same active life style.

The Ten Commandments To Prevent Osteoporosis

1. Eat plenty of calcium-rich foods or take supplements.
2. Limit alcohol, caffeine and soda pop.
3. Avoid fasting diets.
4. Exercise at least four times per week.
5. Take estrogen if you are high risk for osteoporosis.
6. Avoid too much thyroid supplement, it softens the bones.
7. Avoid smoke, either first hand or second hand.
8. Listen to your doctor.
9. Spend less time in your easy chair.
10. Perform weight-bearing activities on your spine such as walking.

Who needs estrogen to help prevent osteoporosis? The medical rule is that estrogen should begin immediately at menopause and continue for at least seven years, since 50 percent of the bone loss occurs in the first seven years after menopause.

How can you reduce your risk of developing delicate bones? Eat a calcium-rich diet, exercise with weight-bearing activities like walking and take estrogen or etidronate after menopause if it is prescribed. Additionally, calcitonin, a hormone is being used in several medical centers across the country to harden the bones. Estrogen with small amounts of testosterone is prescribed by some doctors. Ask your doctor if this would be helpful for you.

*   *   *

Treatment Of Complications Of Spinal Osteoporosis

Bed rest (Maximum three days), pain relief, moist heat.
Assisted ambulation as soon as possible, brace if needed.
Theraputic exercise as soon as pain permits.

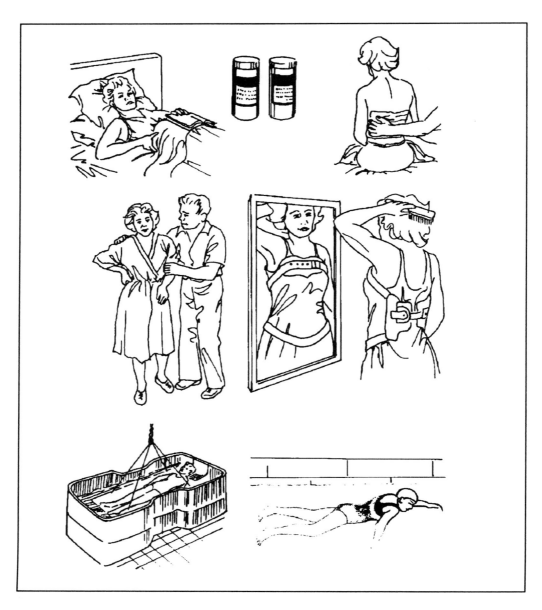

< 8 >

First Aid For Flare Ups—Keeping Active

You can relieve pain from back aches,
then use stretching to stop muscle spasms.

The goal of this chapter is to show the reader how to prevent the chronic pain syndrome from developing after the back has been injured.

Several types of therapy can help relieve inflammation, decrease swelling, improve blood supply and carry away the toxins from the muscles. The first and simplest method is to rest the injured area. To allow complete rest of the back, you should take a cushion from the couch and put it under the sheets on your bed at about the level of your knees.

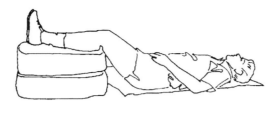

Illustration 80

Illustration 80 shows that the cushion will help support your knees and your hips in a flexed position. This position keeps minimum stress on your low back to allow natural healing. Usually only two or three days of rest are needed. Frequently, the total rest will not be enough to relieve your pains and you will need to take the next step. Use the memory device AIMS to remember: Aspirin, Ice, Massage, Stretching.

Take aspirin or anti-inflammatory medications or use aspirin creams that contain methylsalicylate, a form of aspirin. If you develop an upset stomach from aspirin, you may need to consider taking a different anti-inflammatory medication. None of these medications claim to be superior to aspirin but they may not cause as much stomach distress. Maximum doses of aspirin should not exceed 12 aspirin tables daily for adults. At that dosage, you may have ringing in your ears and that means you are getting some aspirin toxicity and need to decrease the amount of aspirin you take.

Ice—you may or may not choose to use aspirin—but if you have a new injury, you will surely want to know how to use ice therapy. Ice therapy was partially described in a previous chapter, but here are more details. We recommend making an ice lollipop. To make an ice lollipop, freeze water in several styrofoam cups. Remove one cup from the freezer and peel away the top one inch of styrofoam. An alternative way to make an ice lollipop is to freeze water in a styrofoam or plastic cup and put a tongue blade or popsicle stick in the ice. Either way you have a handle to work with. See illustration 81.

Apply the ice in a circular motion over the injured area. Keep the ice moving. After a few minutes it causes an aching sensation. After five minutes there is burning—stop icing for the next two minutes then, repeat the process

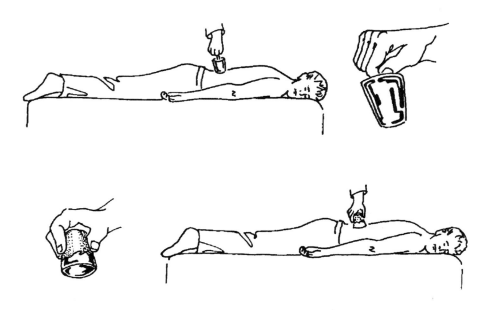

Illustration 81

until numbness develops. The ice temporarily breaks the cycle of pain and spasm and can be repeated three times daily. Remember to massage gently, not deeply.

If your pain is still not relieved by gentle massage or rubbing of the area after using the ice, consider nonprescription anti-inflammatory medications other than aspirin. At present, Ibuprofen is available in several forms of nonprescription strength. These are presented by Advil, Nuprin, Medipren and others with a maximum dose of two tablets every four hours. These are often better tolerated than aspirin but should still be taken with food to protect your stomach lining.

More than any other activity, stretching will stop pain by stopping spasms and muscle tightness. Stretching is the centerstone of pain control. A muscle can't be tight and in spasm while it is being stretched. Specific stretches are demonstrated in Chapter 10.

Daily Activities And Back Pain

As you read along, look closely at the accompanying illustrations to see exactly how the activities are done. These motions are the most efficient for preventing back pain everyday.

1. For reaching, stand on a stool with a slight flex in your knees rather than standing up straight with your arms overhead.

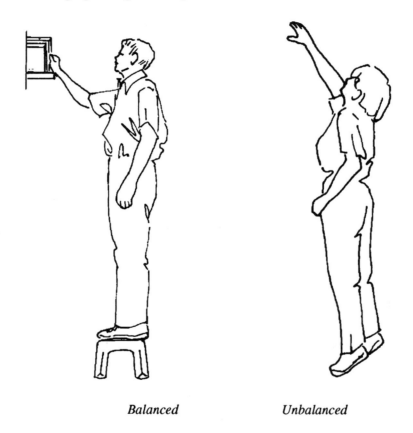

Balanced　　　　*Unbalanced*

Illustration 82

2. When moving heavy objects, push with your body weight rather than pulling them.

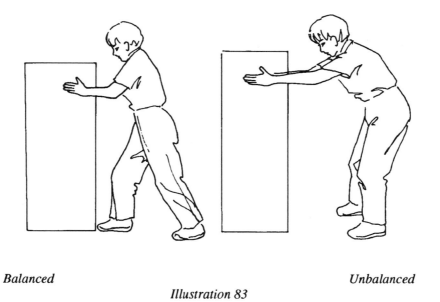

Balanced   *Unbalanced*

Illustration 83

3. To lift a bulky object, drop one knee to the floor, don't squat. Keep the object close to your body when lifting and carrying.

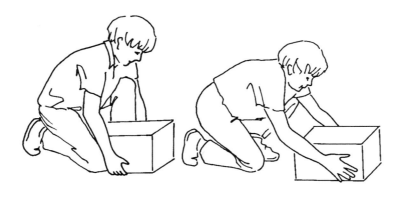

Balanced   *Unbalanced*

Illustration 84

4. When standing for a prolonged time, stand with one foot forward, knees slightly bent and raise one foot and rest it on an object. The drawing at the far left puts strain on the small facet joints of your back. The middle illustration shows how a small stool can help the pain by normalizing the curve of your back. The military stance is too rigid for the low back curve.

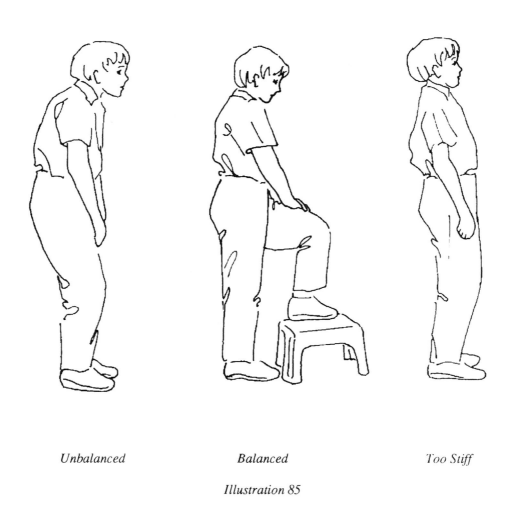

Unbalanced   *Balanced*   *Too Stiff*

Illustration 85

5. When sitting, flex the hips and knees but do not bend forward in the chair. Get your feet under you and rise using the strength of your leg muscles. Don't bend forward to get your body weight over your feet.

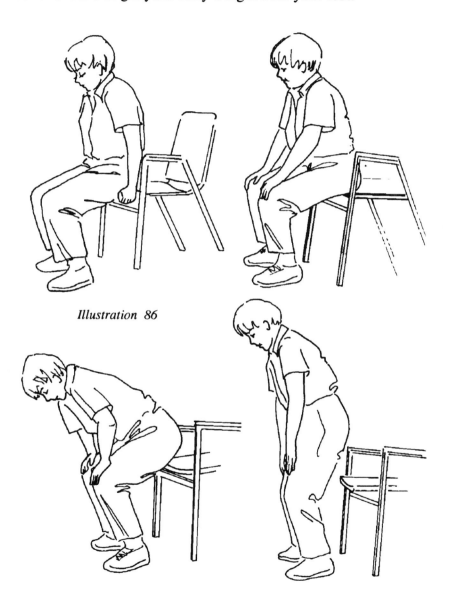

Illustration 86

6. If you are lifting light objects, raise one leg in the air or do a partial squat.

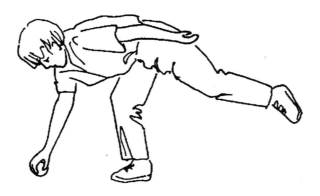

Illustration 87

7. To carry a weight, straighten up slowly, keep the object close to you and shift the weight to your back leg before you start walking.

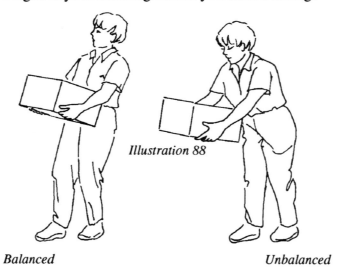

Illustration 88

Balanced   *Unbalanced*

8. If you are trying to vacuum at work, then keep one leg in front of the other. Don't bend in the back to push the vacuum. Preferably, use a light canister vacuum.

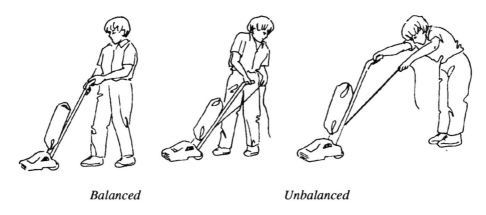

Balanced   *Unbalanced*

Illustration 89

9. When lifting light objects out of the trunk of your car, raise one knee on the bumper, pull the object as close to you as possible, then lift.

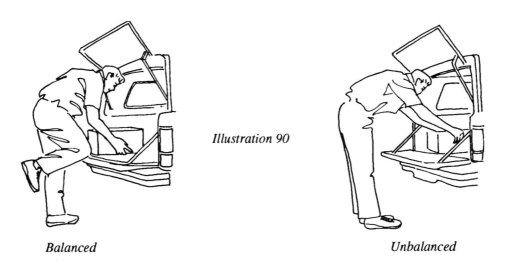

Illustration 90

Balanced   *Unbalanced*

10. When shaving or brushing your teeth, or washing dishes, bend your knees.

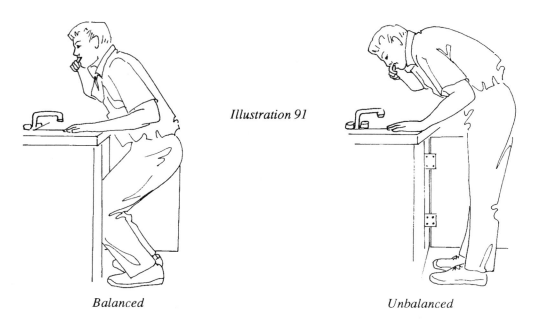

Illustration 91

Balanced   *Unbalanced*

11. When driving an automobile, sit with your back firmly against the car seat and move the seat forward so you have your knees higher than your hips.

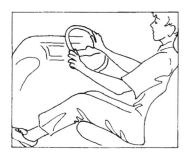

Illustration 92

12. To get into or out of the car, back into the car and once you are on the seat you can lift your legs into position. Reverse this process when leaving the car.

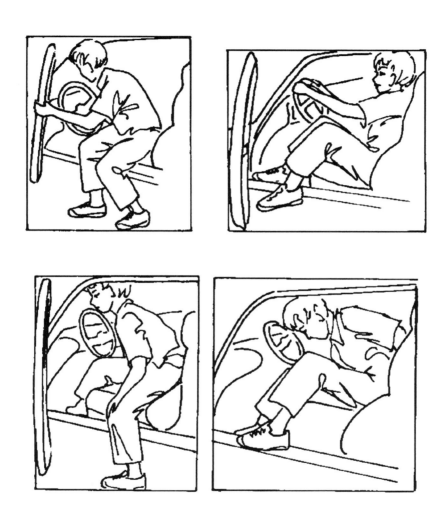

Illustration 93

13. When reaching into the refrigerator or stove or under the sink, go down on one knee to see the item you want. Don't bend and twist to the side.

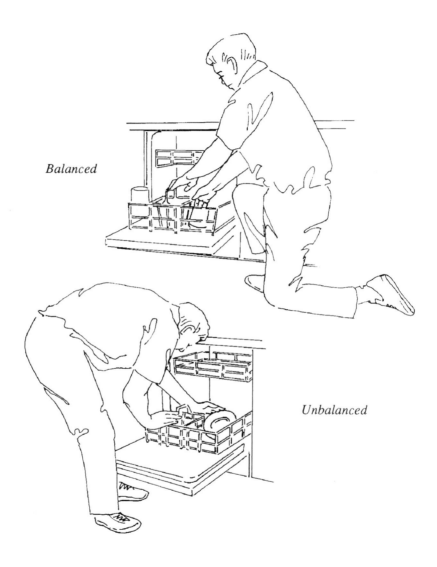

Balanced

Unbalanced

Illustration 94

14. Sitting at work or home often increases pain if not done correctly. Sit slightly reclined with your knees higher than your hips, bring your chair close to your work. Don't bend over the table. It may be helpful to put a small cushion behind your low back or a rolled towel if you need additional support.

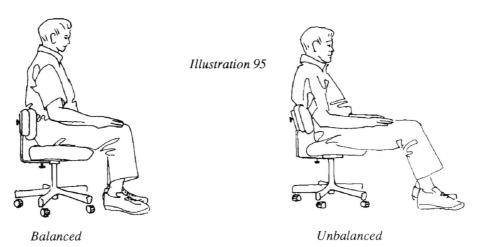

Illustration 95

Balanced   *Unbalanced*

15. Many people bend down to tie the shoe. It is much simpler to bring the shoe up onto a chair and tie it there, or purchase a loafer-type shoe.

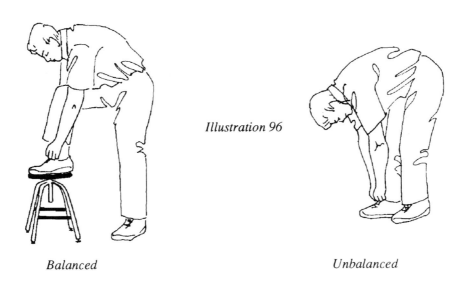

Illustration 96

Balanced   *Unbalanced*

16. If your phone is on a table without a chair, bend your knees to lower yourself to the table level or place a chair near the phone.

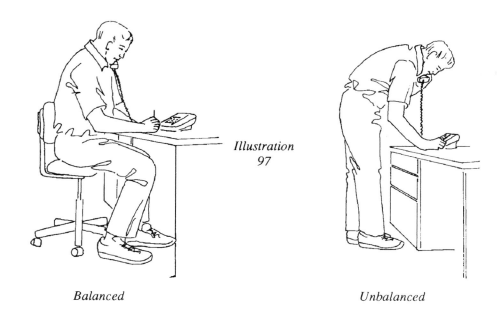

Illustration 97

Balanced　　　　　　　　　　　　　　　　*Unbalanced*

17. When you are washing stains or spills from the floor, position yourself on all fours. Be sure your head is in line with your spine. Put a small cushion or towel under your knees.

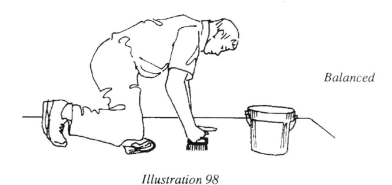

Balanced

Illustration 98

18. Ironing creates problems because it occasionally requires prolonged standing, so raise one foot on a small stool. Be creative, you can find something on which to rest one foot.

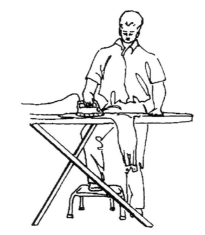

Illustration 99

19. When carrying a suitcase, it's easier to carry two small suitcases rather than carrying one large one.

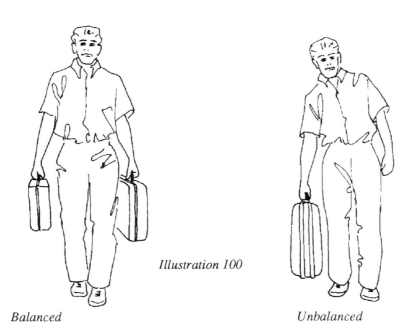

Illustration 100

Balanced   *Unbalanced*

20. For sitting at work. If you have a desk job, search for a comfortable chair with a firm back support. You should be able to adjust the seat to your body keeping your knees even with or higher than your hips. If your chair is too high for your feet to touch the floor comfortably then place a few books under your feet. Be sure to sit on the full chair and not just on the front of the seat. Look for a chair with an adjustable lumbar support. Leaning forward on your chair to work increases the force on your back by about 500 percent.

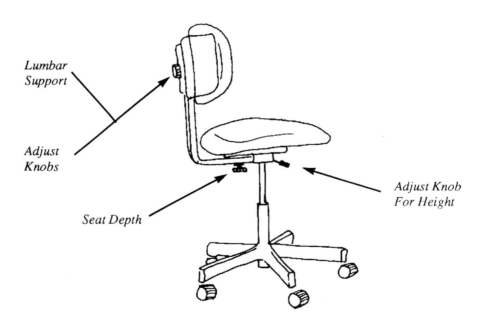

Illustration 101

21. When you retire at night or take a nap, sleep on your side. Keep your bottom leg straightened and bend your upper leg so that it lies in front of you on a pillow. If you have to sleep on your back, place a small flat pillow under your low back to preserve the natural curve of your spine. Place a pillow between your knees when you sleep on your side.

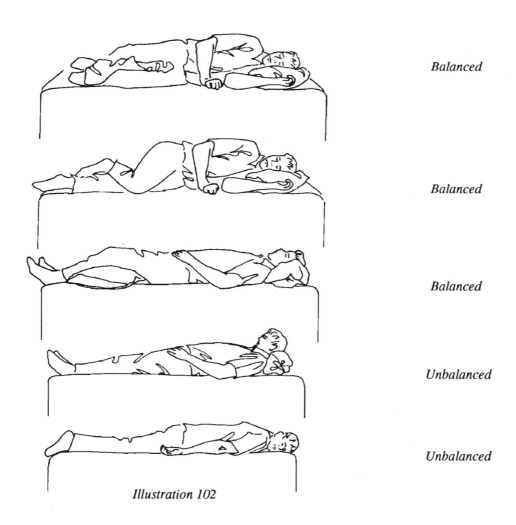

Balanced

Balanced

Balanced

Unbalanced

Unbalanced

Illustration 102

22. To get up from bed, use your hands to press yourself up to a sitting position while swinging your legs over the side of the bed.

Illustration 103

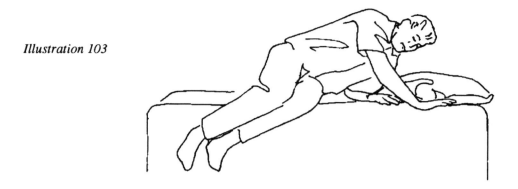

23. If you want to read while you are in bed, use a small flat pillow and place it between the headboard and the small of your back for support.

Illustration 104

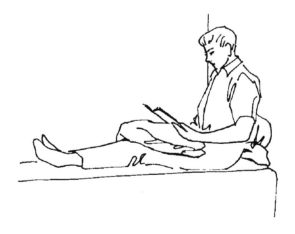

< 9 >

Armor-Plating The Spine

*Toughened muscles will
shield your back from routine injuries.*

"Give me fifty push-ups, mister," ordered the drill sergeant. "Don't even think of resting."

Armor-plating the spine is not an adventure in punishment, the kind of hard instruction you might get in boot camp in the army. Strengthening the spine is a common-sense approach to protecting your back with a program you can do at home. No health club dues or fancy clothes are required unless you wish. Play your favorite music while you warm up for a few minutes and stretch those tight muscles before you begin your back-power exercises.

Your back is enveloped in a shell of flexible, helpful muscles. Just as a radio tower is held up by guy lines on four sides, so your spine must be supported and protected on all four sides. Let's begin with the abdominal or front and side muscles.

You won't have to do boring sit-ups for hours trying to flatten your

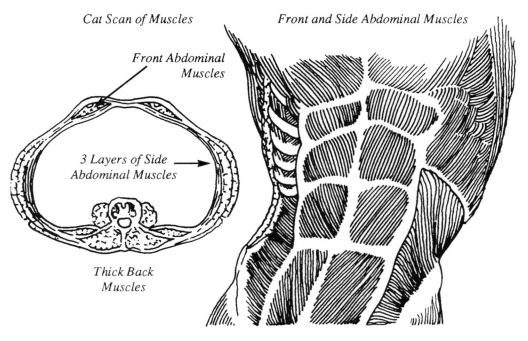

Cat Scan of Muscles   *Front and Side Abdominal Muscles*

Front Abdominal Muscles

3 Layers of Side Abdominal Muscles

Thick Back Muscles

Illustration 105

abdomen to see your toes. Crunches are safer, better, more specific exercises to tone the muscles. As seen in illustration 105, there are four sets of abdominal muscles. However, a simple crunch will bring them all into play in seconds. See illustration 106 for the forward crunch.

From the start position with your back on the floor, flex your knees to take the strain off your back. Next, reach with your hands and put them

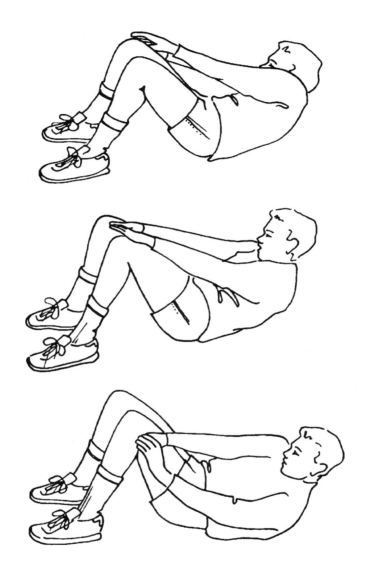

Illustration 106

between your knees. Lie back until your shoulder blades are again touching the floor. Now, reach forward and go to the left of your knees with your hands. Lie back then go forward with your hands to the right of your knees. Focus your eyes on the ceiling above your head so you don't strain your neck while tightening your abdominal muscles.

Ideally, doing ten crunches in each position will tone the abs. (abdominal muscles). Do each crunch slowly and contract your abdominal muscles so you feel a slight burn in them with each upward movement.

Now you're ready to ride a horse. A horse is a small unit you can purchase for use at home or you can use an existing counter or *sturdy* table. Horse is another name for a Roman chair or hyperextension machine—a back strengthening machine. If you have a "horse," then hold onto the "reins" (handles) while you climb on. Tuck your legs under the leg pads. To start, hold onto the handles while you bend your upper body downward. Next, raise your upper body as you feel the muscles contract and tighten in your low and middle back. If your back is weak, this will be quite difficult. Only raise up to a position parallel with the floor. See Illustration 107.

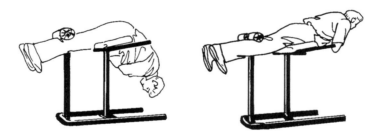

Illustration 107

Work up to three sets of ten repetitions. If this is too difficult, then restrict your movement so that you only go down part way initially. It will get easier with time. If you get dizzy, stop the exercise.

What! You don't have a horse at your house? No problem. You can use the same counter you used for the SAFE back test, the one you took in

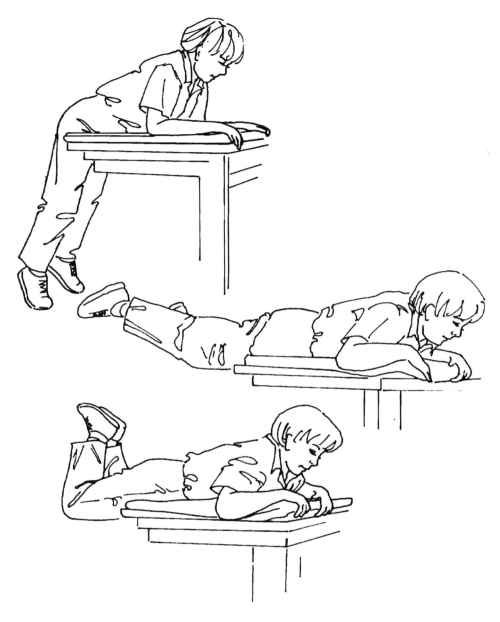

Illustration 108

Chapter 2. Don't worry, you don't need an assistant for this movement.

Lean forward over a counter with a pillow placed beneath your abdomen. See illustration 108. Hold onto the edge or other side of the counter as you lift both legs off the floor and straighten them. At first, this may be quite impossible. It will quickly become easier until you can impress your family.

If this is still too difficult, then assume the same position and bend your knees as far as possible, then lift your legs. See illustration 108. This can be done with less back strength.

Row your back to health. A quiet splash of the oars in the water and the gentle surge of the row boat remind us of a young couple gliding peacefully across a lake. Life's faster pace and new technology have replaced the row boat with Jet Skis and parasailing.

Row boats took advantage of the back muscles and the outing was invigorating as the oars pulled through the water. Strong backs and shoulders were built and helped to prevent future injury. It was fun.

Now you can have a "row boat" for home use. Inexpensive rowing machines utilizing piston-like air chambers to provide resistance are available. See illustration 109. If you want to go the deluxe route, then purchase a rowing machine that uses a flywheel for resistance. These units are very smooth and a pleasure to use.

Illustration 109

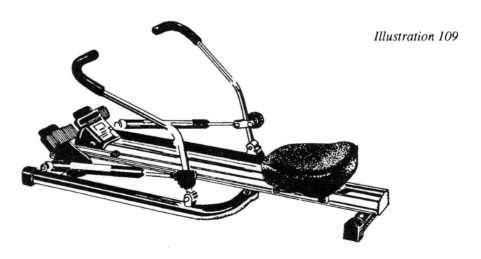

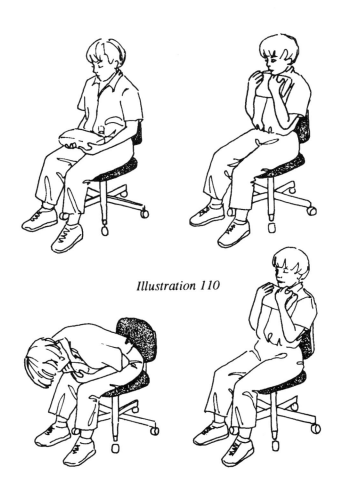

Illustration 110

Start with one minute of rowing. This can be very strenuous if you try to go too fast. Take your time. You didn't get out of shape in one day and you won't reverse your physical condition in one hour.

Rowing is usually done incorrectly. As you hold the handles, push backward with your legs, then pull the handles toward you as you lean backward. Go slow enough that you don't have any back pain. Your back will tell you if you have weak, flabby muscles. Slowly build up the rowing by adding one minute per week. You'll be amazed at your progress after two months. "Two Months!" you say. Yes, it will take that long. When it comes to restoring back strength, it takes time. The time is going to pass anyway, so keep active.

Sugar—20 pounds of it will make you feel great. Sugar—the great soother. Who doesn't like an occasional sweet treat? Now you can keep the sugar in plain sight, ready for your beck and call. There's a catch. You can't open the bag. It must be intact to strengthen your back. How?

Sit on your kitchen chair with the 20-pound bag of sugar sitting in your lap. Now pull the bag of sugar up to your chest with both hands. See illustration 110, for the sequence. Next, lean forward as far as possible or until you feel pain. If you feel pain, then, back off. Now return to the sitting position. Repeat this ten times. Do three sets of ten repetitions. Your back muscles will feel invigorated.

Work at these home exercises. Two months is a good period of time. Look back at your progress. Take the Safe Back Test in Chapter 2 again to monitor your progress. You'll be delighted.

Home exercise is convenient, inexpensive and efficient. What if you are a person who likes to be around a crowd and enjoys companionship while exercising? Then you'll want to go to your local health facility. In the next chapter, we will show you how to strengthen your back without using every machine in the building.

If you want, go ahead and make this a social time. You are welcome to use the equipment. We'll show you what you absolutely need to restore your back without spending two hours a day in the gym.

< 10 >

Building Endurance And Performance

Back exercise machines are designed to stress
muscle groups that strengthen the spine.

So you've decided to go to a health club. The messages your body has been sending of general crankiness, torpor, vague aches and pains, listlessness and fatigue have finally captured your attention. You are ready to do something about yourself. You are going to develop a program that will recondition your body, but you are unfamiliar with the body-building machines waiting for you.

Walking into the gym for the first time will not be as intimidating if you keep an open mind. The home program I've already described will strengthen your spine muscles and restore motion to your aching, stiff back, but the gym will restore endurance and performance. Using the power machines in the gym is like putting a Porsche engine into the first car you ever had. Your back and body will operate most efficiently and with more zest when you strengthen it. Endurance and performance will help you with your tennis game, hiking, aerobics or playing with the kids. You'll see how the spinal engine works. Actually, in this section you'll learn how to bulletproof your back. Your spine is made for motion and activity. When you don't use your spine, it begins to deteriorate. Which machines should you use to help build your spine?

Before I describe the different machines, it's important for you to understand the term Spinal Engine—this was coined by Panjabi, an exercise physiologist. It demonstrates how to excel at physical performance by using the muscles and the ligaments of the trunk. As a golfer takes a back swing, his trunk muscles tighten and in the process stretch the fascia or shrink-wrap around the muscles while the ligaments and tendons of the back, rib cage and shoulders stretch and tighten. Like a stretched rubber band. This triple action is then reversed by the swing at the golf ball. The tightened tissues including tendons, ligaments and fascia act like a sling shot to increase performance as they spring back. The "follow through" in tennis, baseball, handball, completes the motion cycle of the spinal engine and lets the force of your swing dissipate gently.

Walking, running and swimming take advantage of the spinal engine in optimum performance. Once you are aware of the spinal engine, you can increase your performance in the activities of daily living. Getting out of a chair, carrying groceries from the trunk of the car to the house, vacuuming and yard work can all be performed more easily when your spinal engine is "tuned."

Most back pain is caused by weakened back muscles and unpredictable movements of the vertebra due to this instability. In Chapter 2 we discussed back strength. Men should have 120 percent of their body weight as back strength while women should have 100 percent of their body weight as back strength. By using the specialized trunk machines described in this chapter and a few other pieces of equipment in a gym, you can restore the function to your back.

Before you start on any machines, first warm up for five minutes on a stationary bike to increase the joint fluids, and thicken the cartilage pads in the joints. Next, stretch using the flexion and extension stretches.

Now you are ready. What do you do next? You ask for a personal trainer for a few sessions to learn how to use the machines properly to obtain the most benefit without injury. Start with a comfortable weight. Don't force it. You have plenty of time to fix your back for your future. Which machines do you need to use to strengthen your back?

1. A back extension machine.
2. An abdominal machine.
3. A leg press.
4. A leg extension.
5. A leg curl.
6. A rotary torso.
7. A pullover.

I use Nautilus in this example since it is a product which is probably best known and used in fitness centers nationwide. Now turn back to the C.A.T. scan of the back and abdominal muscles shown on page 124. We want to optimize the function of each of these muscle groups and to do that I recommend using machines for the first two months until you have stabilized the muscles around your spine. Then, you can proceed to use free weights if you desire.

Back Extension Machine. Tune up your spinal engine. This machine works by stabilizing your pelvis with a seat belt while your feet are fixed against a foot pad. You push against a padded bar with your back muscles. Go slowly. Push back for two to three seconds through the entire range of motion, and when you reach the maximum motion, come forward slowly. Take twice as long to come forward as it takes you to push backward. You'll increase strength quickly in this manner. Avoid throwing your weight into the machine; move slowly and precisely.

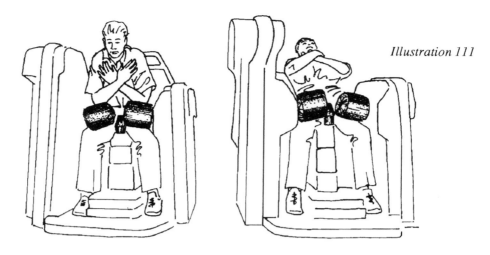

Illustration 111

Back Extension Machine

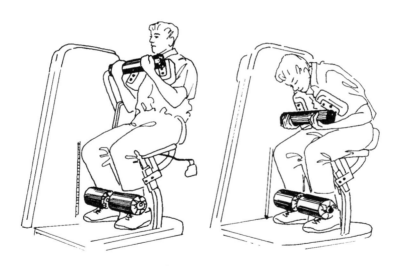

Abdominal Machine

Illustration 112

Abdominal Machine. You want to strengthen the front abdominal muscles to help them act as a brace for your spine for the activities of daily living. Always start with the lightest weight. Work up until you can do three sets of ten repetitions easily before moving to the next weight. You are not trying to win a contest. Work for slow, steady progress. See illustration 112 for the motion.

Leg Extension. Strong legs will help to protect your back during lifting activities. The leg extension will give you strong thigh muscles to assist you with lifting safely while protecting your back. See the beginning and final motions in illustration 113. If you have knee problems, ask your doctor or therapist how best to strengthen these muscles.

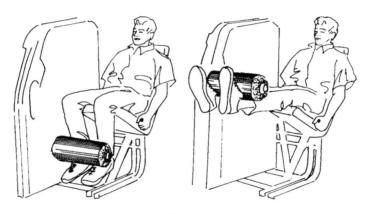

Leg Extension

Illustration 113

Leg Press. This machine always looks like a macho exercise but don't let it fool you. It strengthens all the muscles of the thigh and buttock and it helps them work as a functional unit. The muscles are large and must be strong so the weight you use will be higher for this machine than for most of the other machines. Watch the motion. Two seconds pushing, then four seconds to return to the beginning position. Feel the muscles work. Perform three sets of ten repetitions to gain maximum benefit. Illustration 114.

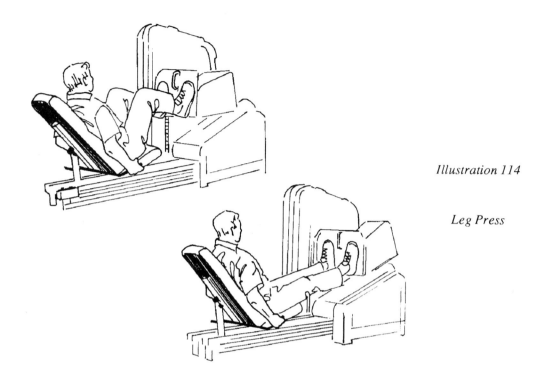

Illustration 114

Leg Press

Leg Curl. To isolate and strengthen the hamstring muscles this machine is excellent. Move smoothly. Initially, you will be able to lift only a few pounds using this machine but with time, your strength will increase. If you feel exhausted muscles from this machine, then lower the weights. Again, three sets of ten repetitions will help build endurance. Illustration 115.

Pullover. This unique machine works the abdominal and chest muscles in a smooth rhythmic motion. If you have shoulder problems, then avoid this machine or use one with a range limiting device that allows for protected, limited movement of the shoulders. Ask your therapist or certified trainer for help if you have shoulder problems. Most people love this machine and the way it makes them feel as it stretches and strengthens the muscles.

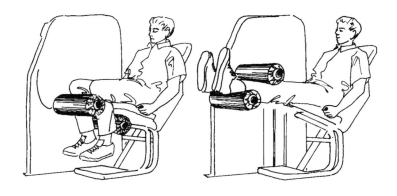

Leg Curl

Illustration 115

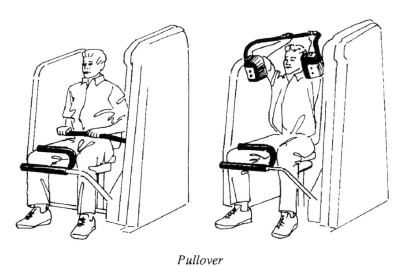

Pullover

Illustration 116

Pull down for two seconds and return to the starting position in four seconds. If you can't perform three sets of ten repetitions, don't be frustrated; keep working, it will come in a few more weeks. See illustration 116.

Rotary Torso. This machine works an integral part of your spinal engine. The motion will stabilize the side abdominal and small spine muscles. This machine is used last—after you've reached about 80 percent of your back strength. Don't start with the rotary torso until the fourth or fifth week of your strengthening program or you'll have more pain. Do the gentle rotary stretches in place of the machine for the first month. When you do begin, start with the lowest weights and move slowly. Consider this machine as the icing on the cake.

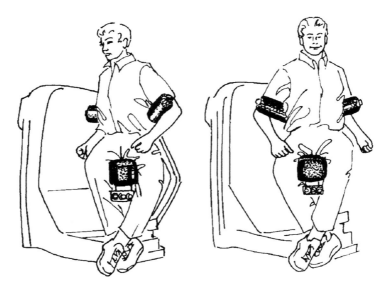

Rotary Torso

Illustration 117

What, is that all? What about all the other machines in the club?

The program we have designed strengthens and protects your spine. It's not a program to strengthen your biceps or win contests. Our goal is to give you back the ability to take control of your life by restoring your spine to good health. If you wish to use other machines then do so after the eight week program is completed and your back function is near normal.

The basics in this chapter help you recover your back health one day at a time. Remember—the maximum number of strengthening workouts in a week is three, one every other day. If you try to strengthen your back every day, then your muscles will not have time to recover and you will have additional problems with fatigue and pain.

However, stretch twice every day to keep the healing, growing muscles flexible. I wish you every success in the recovery of your former self. Keep at it. You can do it.

< 11 >

Stretching Stops Pain

The household cat knows how to flex rest-softened muscles,
making them relax.

Watching a youngster perform the splits or seeing a student fold his legs and sit in the lotus position might make you cringe. And you might wonder what is the secret of baseball great Nolan Ryan who looks and functions at an age level twenty years younger than he is. Come to think of it, how did Mary Lou Retton win her Olympic medals? Are these people different than you are? Do they have some magic formula for staying and feeling young in their muscles?

The answers to these questions and why you feel stiff in the morning may astound you. Look out your back window and watch a cat when it gets up from a nap. Instinctively, it stretches to ready the muscles for action.

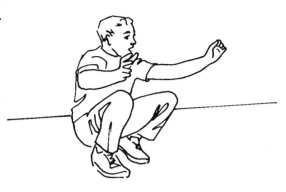

Children squat down any time to observe an insect in the grass and may stay in that position for minutes a a time. See illustration 118. Most adults fall backward when they try to do this. Why?

Illustration 118

Rest-softened muscles become stiff and tight. Just as children had to be "taught" to sit still, adults must be retaught to get moving. "Unless you become as little children, you shall not enter the kingdom of heaven." Wise words from the Good Book. Feel the joys and excitement of life that children feel. Learn to waken the sleeping child within you with flexible muscles. It's possible. Here's how.

Stretching and relaxation are synonymous. A stretched muscle is relaxed. A relaxed muscle is not tight and painful. How are you supposed to do this? You can't go out in the yard and roll around or the neighbors will begin to wonder about you. Two simple ideas will help.

First, most cities and towns have established exercise trails. These are safe, well-lit areas where stretching is encouraged with signs placed at intervals. Usually these "trails" are located within parks in a peaceful surrounding. The trail gives you a good overall workout at the intensity that is perfect for you.

If you live in the Midwest, winters may make this outdoor stretching a life-threatening experience. If so, you can have your own "home park and trail." We'll concentrate on the home park.

But first, you have to agree that stiffness of muscles is your responsibility. A therapist can stretch your muscles passively but cannot adequately stretch the tiny muscles located between the vertebrae and the spine protective muscles which cause much of the stiffness. Therapists can teach you how to be responsible for your back to prevent you from becoming dependent on the medical system. To keep flexible, make it fun!

S-T-R-E-T-C-H-I-N-G—the very word is an action word. Entire books are written about stretching but you only need perform the basic stretches to keep your back in action. All you need is a flat surface and a little space. This is your home park. Adjust the lighting and put on your favorite music or watch TV.

Start with a warm up. Walk a few minutes, go up and down the stairs five times, or use a small trampoline or bicycle to start the blood pumping. Stiff muscles need plenty of oxygen-rich blood to oil them.

Thera-Band Shoulder Stretch

"Reach for the sky, pardner." Cowboys were especially good at following this instruction when a gun was poked in their back. But you can relax as you perform this stretch in the quiet atmosphere of your home. This brief stretch will give you an idea of your upper body flexibility. See illustration 120. Keep your elbows locked and straight and move slowly. Never force a stretch. Stretch for pleasure not for pain. Use a longer towel to begin. As you become more flexible, use a shorter towel. Do this ten times. This will take about one half minute.

Knee To Chest—The Fetal Position

To feel younger, you must act younger. This movement will stretch your low back and hip muscles. Lie on your back on the floor. First pull one knee to your chest, then the other. Finally, pull both knees to the chest and hold for thirty seconds. If you feel pain, then back off. Stretching should not be a forced activity. See illustration 16 on page 18.

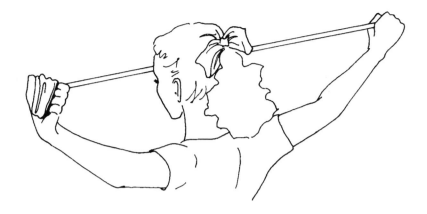

Illustration 120

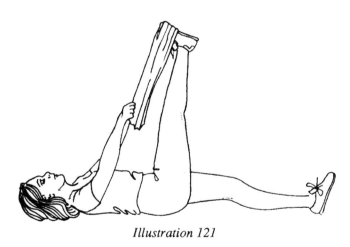

Illustration 121

Hamstring Stretch — The Most Important Stretch

Place yourself on your back as in the illustration 121. Place a towel around your foot and keeping your knee straight, pull your foot toward the midday sun. Repeat with the other leg. Hold thirty seconds.

Standing. This may be easier for you. Place one heel on a pedestal (a chair or counter). Many people start with a low pedestal and raise it as their flexibility increases. These muscles are important for protecting your back when you bend forward. If your hamstrings are too tight, your back will need to bend more when you bend forward. Save your back, stretch your legs.

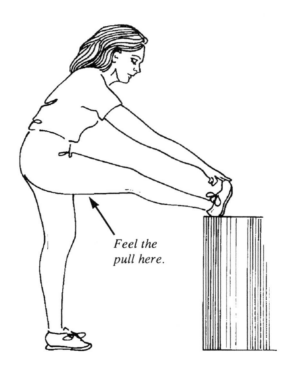

Feel the pull here.

Illustration 122

Gluteal Stretch

Those powerful muscles on the buttocks are often ignored with the result of an overworked back. The gluteals help the back lift you to a standing position from bending forward. As you stretch this area, you will be keenly aware of a muscle group you forgot existed. Lie on the floor with your knees bent as much as possible. Cross your right leg over your left knee. See illustration 123. Pull up your left knee toward your body. At first you will have very little motion. These gluteals have become shortened from disuse. Give them time, they'll become supple. Repeat with the opposite side. Hold for thirty seconds.

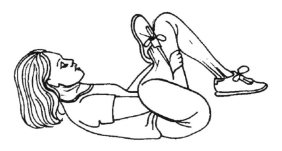

Illustration 123

Helicopter

This stretch was named for a particularly aggressive Type A patient who couldn't move slowly for any activity. He would generate a wind in the therapy area until we finally retrained him to understand that stretching is a gentle exercise.

Sit on the floor or on a chair without arms. See illustration 124. With a wooden closet rod across the shoulders, turn slowly until the tip of the stick passes your nose. Don't force it. Passing by your nose is a goal that most people reach after two or three weeks. One side will be stiffer than the other. Twist fifty times to each side.

Most people become addicted to this exercise. After a few days,

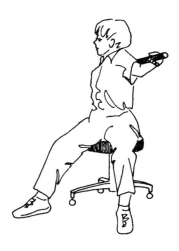

Illustration 124

stiffened muscles in the mid to low back give up their spasm while clicks and pops occur in the spine as frozen, stiff vertebrae once again start moving.

When To Extend Yourself

Just as the power cord to a super computer is protected by a flexible, waterproof, impact-resistant rubber tubing, your spinal cord is encased in a flexible, impact-resistant bony tube called the spine. The "wiring" in your spine is much more complex than that of a super computer. Here's a way to recondition and protect your wiring while keeping the spine supple.

This flexible tube can't stretch itself so you must stretch the muscles around the tube to keep it freely moving. In the following exercise, the spine actually lengthens and produces a form of individual traction.

Lie on your stomach on the floor. See illustration 125. Lift up on to your elbows while keeping your hips on the floor. Hold thirty seconds. If this is easy, then lift up until your elbows are straight and your back is arched more. See illustration 126. Try to keep your hips on the floor. AVOID PAIN.

Illustration 125

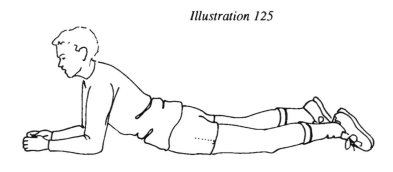

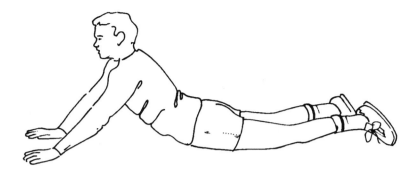

Illustration 126

Alternate Arm And Leg

A greater challenge, this exercise strengthens as it stretches and will make your muscles tingle or burn. Lie on the floor face down. Straighten your arms and legs. See illustration 127. Raise your right arm and left leg and hold for ten seconds. Repeat three times. Rest a few seconds. Now do the same with the opposite arm and leg. Now you're ready for the:

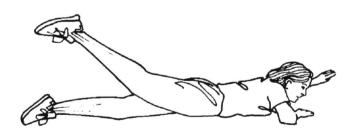

Illustration 127

Superstretch

Lie on the floor in the same position. Raise both arms and both legs with elbows and knees locked in the straight position. See illustration 128. Feel the pull throughout your back and shoulders. Hold ten seconds, repeat three times. This is the most difficult of all stretches as it includes strengthening at the same time. Now you are ready for some easy ones.

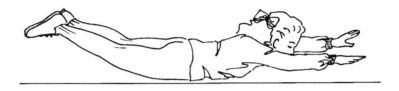

Illustration 128

The Cat

When a cat rises from a lying or resting position, it stretches two ways. First it flexes its back, then arches it's back. See illustration 129. This is a gentle stretch you will enjoy. When on your knees and hands, arch your back and hold for a second then bend your back as you see in illustration 130. Do this ten times in each direction.

Stretching is nature's way of keeping muscles loose and ready for action. These loose muscles do not injure easily. Learn from the animals—stretch before activity. A few minutes of stretching before work or play reduces injury by 90 percent. Flexible, strong muscles rarely become injured. Most back injuries involve soft tissue damage; muscles, ligaments and tendons are damaged. These structures can be kept supple with stretches.

A simple stretch can prevent months of agonizing back pain but more importantly, it can improve your day to day performance. Old people who fall often cannot get up by themselves. They have lost flexibility and strength. This does not need to happen. Minimal effort produces results when it comes to stretching. Age is not a deterrent, impatience and neglect are.

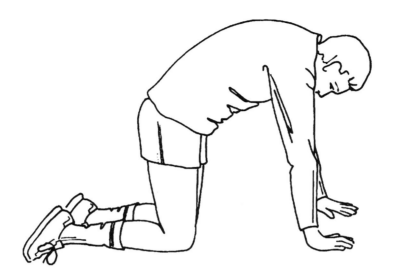

Illustration 129

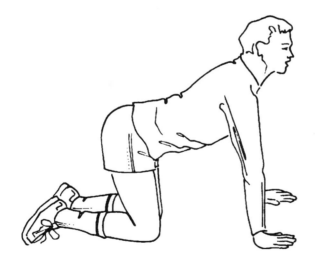

Illustration 130

< 12 >

Aerobics

*Creating strength, flexibility and endurance through
exercises that increase heart rate.*

Smell the fragrance after a heavy rain. Take in deep breaths of oxygen-rich air. When you fill your lungs with air, you are literally defining the meaning of Aerobics—"with oxygen". Your muscles must be bathed in oxygen in order to function at peak capacity. Oxygen gives injured muscles the power to heal and "stale" muscles the ability to waken and develop their full potential. As we become better "trained", our bodies become more efficient at extracting oxygen from the blood. The weekend athlete is a good example of inappropriate motion. For five days each week, he sits in an office or has a sedentary job. On Saturday he jumps on his bicycle and rides thirty miles. Sunday, Monday and Tuesday he's stiff and sore. He hasn't learned to "listen to his body". He exercises too hard, too infrequently and exercises *anerobically* without adequate oxygen. Exercise at this high intensity produces activity in different enzyme systems. They come into play because there is not enough oxygen for the muscles.

Later, muscle stiffness results from the build up of acids and other chemicals in the muscles. Moderation is the key to healthy exercises.

Anerobic exercise is inefficient and without adequate oxygen during periods of physical stress, the muscles begin to "burn".

This "burn" made our bicyclist slow down until he caught up aerobically. If he had ridden aerobically (with oxygen) at a slightly slower pace, he could have pedalled without his muscles paying the price. The question then is: If being a weekend athlete is not enough, how much exercise is sufficient?

Your heart requires twenty minutes of aerobic exercise three times per week at 80 percent of your maximum heart rate. What is 80 percent of your maximum heart rate (MHR)? It is easily calculated by subtracting your age from 220. if you are 30 years old, then subtract 30 from 220: 220 - 30 = 190, your maximum heart rate. Eighty percent of your maximum heart rate is 152: 190 x 80 percent = 152. So twenty minutes at 152 beats per minute three times weekly is the *minimum* amount of exercise your heart needs to function efficiently if you are 30 years old.

Very few people should begin exercise at 80 percent of their maximum heart rate. Developing muscles need more time to rebuild "sleepy" fibers to function optimally. If you are out of shape aerobically based on the test in Chapter Two, then start gently. Start for five minutes daily at 40 percent of your maximum heart rate. If you're 40 years old, then 220 - 40 = 180; 180 is your maximum heart rate. 180 x 40 percent = 72 beats per minute. Add one minute of exercise every three days and work up to at least twenty minutes.

After two weeks, increase to 50 percent of your maximum heart rate: 220 - 40 years old = 180 beats per minute. One hundred eighty times 50 percent = 90 beats per minute. Every two weeks, increase your heart rate by 10 percent: 220 - 40 = 180. One hundred eighty times 60 percent = 108 beats per minute. In four more weeks you are at 80 percent of your maximal heart rate: 220 - 40 = 180, or 180 x 80 percent = 144 beats per minute.

Exercising and a life of movement are a process. As you continue to exercise, you will form more and deeper grooves of memory called engrams. If you are trying to build a house, you must first build a foundation. For any back program to be effective, you need a foundation. Aerobics is only one cornerstone of this foundation. The other three cornerstones are: strength of muscles, flexibility of muscles, and endurance of muscles.

HOW TO CHECK YOUR PULSE

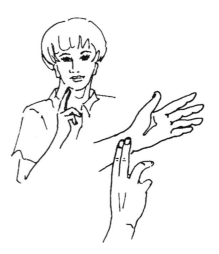

The calculations for a training heart rate are useless unless you can tell approximately what your pulse rate is. Your carotid pulse in the neck can be easily palpated or the wrist pulse is also simple to find. See illustration 131. Count the pulse for six seconds and multiply that number by ten to see how many beats per minute your pulse is. If you count ten beats in six seconds, then multiply the 10 beats x 10 for the number of beats in one minute, which is 100. Pulse meters for the wrist or fingers can be helpful.

Illustration 131

What if you don't have a pulse meter and/or don't want one? Is there an easy way to gauge your heart rate? Yes, thanks to the Borg Scale of perceived exertion. It measures how hard you feel like you are working. This scale runs from six through twenty. Six represents the amount of exertion you feel at rest with a heart rate of about sixty. Below is a slight variation of the Borg Scale to simplify calculating your pulse:

Borg Scale of Perceived Exertion: Number x 10	Verbal Description Of Perceived Effort
6	The amount of exertion you feel at rest.
7	*Very, very light* exertion, like moving about the kitchen.
8	
9	*Very light exertion* like a walk to the mailbox.
10	
11	*Fairly light* exertion like shopping in a mall while carrying a package.
12	
13	*Somewhat hard exertion* like walking upstairs.
14	
15	*Hard exertion* like jogging uphill.
16	
17	*Very hard exertion* like digging a ditch.
18	
19	*Very, very hard* like pushing a car uphill.
20	

Only the odd numbers in the scale are filled in so you can put your own ideas for exertion in the scale. As the exercise intensity increases, your heart rate also increases.

Multiply the number you see by 10 to determine your perceived scale of exertion and your estimated heart rate. Take for example, the exertion required by going for a walk on an incline. If you feel like your effort in walking is somewhat hard, look to the left of the chart at the number 13, which corresponds to "Somewhat hard". Multiply this number by ten to get your estimated pulse rate. Your approximate pulse rate is 130 beats per minute.

The Borg Scale is named after the Swedish exercise physiologist Gunnar Borg who developed it in the 1950s. It is used throughout the world for cardiac rehabilitation to help patients become aware of their perceived effort. These patients have had heart attacks and now are looking for a better, healthier lifestyle. Begin now instead of waiting for a problem to develop. Try using this scale during exercise. Cut it out of the book and carry it with you. Make a smaller copy and plasticize it at the library to keep it waterproof. You'll develop an *exercise engram*.

EVERYBODY NEEDS AN EXERCISE ENGRAM

What is an engram? An engram is a familiar groove of memory in the brain. As an example, we all have an engram for walking. If you see a friend at a distance, you may recognize her by her walk before you can see her face. She may have her head slightly bent forward with arms swinging away from her sides and with hunched shoulders.

Each of us has a personal engram for every activity we perform. Take for example, the TV engram. This is one of our strongest engrams. Many of us come home, eat dinner, then move to the living or television room and watch TV for the evening. As the commercials appear, you may get up and get a snack or go to the bathroom. You do this at a predictable rate. If your television breaks you may actually experience withdrawal as strong as that associated with drugs. The TV engram becomes so ingrained within us that if we usually snack during each commercial, we get almost uncontrolled urges to eat at that time, even when we are not hungry. In a situation like this, you actually need to make new engrams but you can't do it sitting in front of the television. You need to sit in a different chair or in a different room or take up a new activity. If you sit down in your TV chair with the TV turned on you will fall into the old familiar engram of eating. Make yourself some new engrams of exercise.

You might say "I don't feel coordinated when I'm trying a new exercise." Of course not. Your brain doesn't have any engram or groove of memory to look back on. We're not born with coordination, we develop it. When you watch little league or Tee Ball games, you notice that the five and six-year-olds can barely hit a baseball sitting on a two-foot-high tee. They have no memory groove. By the end of their first season in three months, they can hit a slowly pitched ball.

Any of the exercises in this back book can be learned. We all feel uncoordinated when we start a new activity. Think of the first time you tried to hit a golf ball or roll a strike with a bowling ball. It looked easy when others did it so you tried and were disappointed. Don't be discouraged. As you develop exercise engrams you'll feel more comfortable every day. The strength of engrams is increased by repetition. Keep pushing yourself to succeed with this program. The results will astound you.

What determines your overall level of function? It is the *pacemaker in the brain*. Using extreme examples, Olympic sprinters have fast-twitch muscles, muscles that contract very quickly. Ultra-marathoners, people who run 50 or 100 mile races have slow twitch fibers, muscles that contract slowly but have prolonged endurance. You can't change your muscle fiber type but you can learn to take control of the muscles you have.

The pacemaker in your brain is a series of exercise engrams. If you warmed up, stretched and ran a mile every day, you'd be pretty consistent in the amount of time it would take you to cover the distance. The speed of your muscle contractions makes a difference as to whether you're world class or an average runner, but your brain decides how hard your muscles should work.

As you start stretching for your mile run, your brain begins searching for a memory groove that is consistent with this activity. It will quickly find the engram for the one mile run. Then your brain will tell you how hard to run based on past experience. If you want to establish a new level of performance, here is how to do it:

Run your mile and when you're half way, use the Borg Scale of perceived exertion to see where your heart rate is. Your exercise feels like *hard work*. You discover your rate corresponds to number 15 on the Borg Scale. Multiply 15 x 10 and you have your approximate heart rate of 150 beats per minute. If that is less than 80 percent of your maximal heart rate, and you've been following the program, then you can increase your effort to 16 or 17 on the BORG Scale where the effort of exertion feels *very hard*.

This corresponds to a heart rate of 160 to 170 per minute. Only by pushing yourself can you increase your effort. As soon as your mind wanders to your plans for the day or to another topic, your old engram will take over and put you on autopilot at 150 beats per minute. Pick your level of comfort on the Borg Scale and when you are ready, push yourself to the next level.

Aerobics is an integral part of your back rehabilitation. Rehabilitation is functional restoration. By restoring function, we optimize our performance. As our performance reaches normal standards, the back pain usually decreases.

< 13 >

Age Vigorously Or Age Rapidly

*Older people are proving fitness
can improve longevity and physical agility.*

Television is said to be a reflection of society's attitudes. Until recently, it has painted a bleak picture of the elderly, sitting in a rocker or swing on the front porch trying to catch a summer breeze while watching the younger folks pass by. The most exercise these seniors, or masters as we'll call them, received was to raise an arm to wave as young parents ambled by pushing a new baby in a stroller.

But wait, here is the same elderly couple paddling a rubber kayak in an alpine lake. They backpacked their gear two miles in and 2,000 feet up Zigzag mountain in Oregon for a camping, hiking and fishing weekend. They decided to enjoy an active life with their children and grandchildren. There is more to life than dull, desperate days in front of the TV.

Ball State University in Indiana has published research on strength in the elderly—inactive people in nursing homes. In 12 weeks with mild exercises they were able to increase their strength by 300 percent. Those who stopped exercising returned to the weakened state while the exercise group continued to show improvement in strength. In Chapter 14, you'll find more

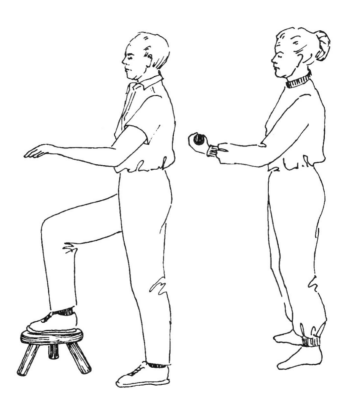

Elderly becoming active again.

Illustration 132

information about strength training for older people.

If nursing home clients can increase their strength as much or more than 300 percent, then you can increase your strength to allow you to fully participate in life.

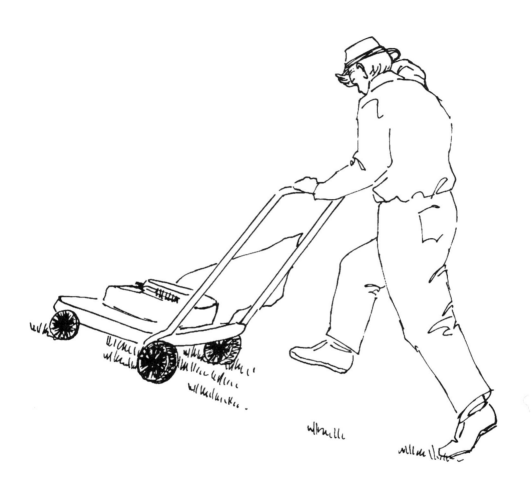

Illustration 133

Have you noticed that the kitchen chairs are heavier than they used to be and the lawn mower is getting harder to push? That old aluminum ladder now feels like it is made out of lead. This deterioration is not inevitable. Why wear out slowly like an old battery sapped of power? Turn your body into a rechargeable battery. I'll show you how to recharge yourself with a graded program. I start with the basics of aerobics, strength, flexibility and endurance then progress slowly as your muscles take on a Lazarus-like quality and come back to life. (See charts following page 167.)

If you're satisfied with the creaking rocker on the front porch, that's fine but if you want to participate with the rest of the active world and share it with friends and loved ones, read on. Take The SAFE back test in Chapter 2. I know it takes effort, but so does everything that is worthwhile. Add your total points up here. If 100 points are possible, see where you fall on the pain to performance scale.

```
Pain_____Performance
 0    10   20   30   40   50   60   70   80   90   100
```

Before you can succeed at any exercise program, you need to have enough oxygen to pump to the muscles. Aerobics is the key. Chapter 11 shows how to build aerobic endurance. Work at this for six weeks then take the variation of the Bruce treadmill test. Dr. R. A. Bruce in his 1970 *Manual Of Exercise Testing* developed this test to set a standard for a progressive program for challenging the heart with exercise. This test is used throughout the world.

Page 166 shows the protocol and speeds necessary to make this test accurate. You also need access to a treadmill with adjustable speed and elevation controls. Ask your doctor to perform this test if you have been a smoker, have other medical problems, a family history of heart disease or are taking any medications. Get your doctor's permission before taking this test. Only your doctor knows any medical problems you may have.

Check your pulse every half minute while on the treadmill using the pulse checking techniques on page 152. Follow the protocol until you reach 80 percent of your maximum heart rate. Record the minutes and seconds.

An active individual exercises aerobically at least three times per week for 20 minutes or more. A sedentary person exercises aerobically less than 20 minutes three times weekly. For example: if you are an active woman and are 30 years old, exercise until you reach 80 percent of your maximum heart rate. Using the active woman chart, draw a line from the age to the numbers of minutes you achieved on the treadmill until you reached 80 percent of your maximum heart rate. Now draw a line from that number on the right through the fitness point. The line intersects with your functional age on the left of the graph. If your functional age is older than your actual age, then you need to increase your aerobic exercise.

If you are a 53-year old sedentary man, exercise until you reach 80 percent of your maximum heart rate. Take the number from the table provided. Using the sedentary graph, draw a line from your age to the number of minutes you exercised to achieve 80 percent of your maximum heart rate. Now draw a line from the number of minutes of exercise on the right of the graph through the fitness point. This line intersects on the left side of the chart with your functional age. If your chronological age and your functional age are the same, then one line will be on the top of the other.

Here is how to determine your aerobic condition: The first line drawn from left to right, from years of age to minutes of duration, will pass through your functional aerobic impairment. Plus (+) numbers mean you are or out of shape. Minus(-) numbers mean you are in good aerobic condition.

I have enclosed a chart to help you calculate your maximum heart rate in a simple fashion. Take 80 percent of the rate as your goal. If you exceed your maximum heart rate or if you stay on the treadmill longer after you reach 80 percent of your maximum heart rate, the test is invalid. Your functional age is based on reaching 80 percent of your maximal heart rate only. If your performance was less than you hoped, then work on building aerobic capacity and endurance and retake the test in one or two months. It's a pleasure to watch and feel your body respond to the program with increased strength, flexibility and endurance. You'll feel and function at a younger age level.

Don't take aging sitting down! Regardless of your level of fitness everyone ages. But fitness makes a world of difference in how people age and what level of function they retain. All animals become less active as they become older including humans, and unfortunately physical capabilities diminish the less active people are.

Take back your independence. No one wants to be dependent on his children or relatives when he is older. Start now. Begin an active program of life fitness and activity.

Here is the brief story of a woman who injured her back and discovered how much out of condition she was. Physically, she was older than her years.

Marjorie worked in the kitchen of a nursing home. She loved the people and catered to them. During a busy lunch time clean-up, she slipped on the watery, greasy floor and landed on her buttocks with a jolt of electricity shooting up through her spine. She suffered compression injuries to several discs with tears of the circular fibers, but no herniation. The tears in the discs caused inflammatory chemicals to be released which caused swelling and pain in her back.

Marjorie had physical therapy with stretching, hot packs and ultrasound which helped the pain but she could not return to work. Finally,

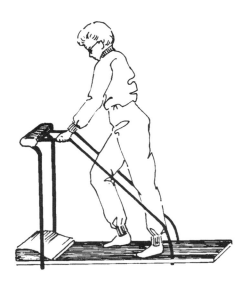

she was referred to rehabilitation with an increasing intensity of strength training of her trunk and legs using machines like the ones in Chapter 10. Because of a family history of heart disease, Marjorie was given a cardiac treadmill before starting her rehabilitation. She lasted three minutes before her heart reached 80 percent of its maximum which gave her a functional age of *90 years*.

In rehabilitation, her strength and movement returned to normal and she was released to work. Marjorie's interests were in the areas of reading and watching movies. Each day after work she cuddled into her favorite recliner and spent the next five or six hours snacking and fantasizing the lives of movie stars and book heroines. Her fitness level slowly deteriorated until she woke up stiff and in severe pain with her back problem gnawing at her with every heart beat. She started exercising again and the pain resolved.

Marjorie's story is repeated thousands of times every day. She was more prone to injury since she was inactive and functionally much older than her chronological 45 years. She took longer to recover because of her life style. Her inactivity caused a decreased blood supply to the discs in her back as well as loss of strength of the muscles and ligaments. Her injury could have been much less severe and she could have healed more quickly had she taken better care of herself.

Age vigorously or age rapidly. Aging is inevitable but aging can be delayed or slowed with a regular program of fitness and strengthening. Oregon's famous body builder, Bill Pearl, has aged gracefully. He starts his day with exercise and eats correctly. He thinks health, has a high quality to his life and is able to perform most activities because he is aging gracefully. If we work at it, we can all age gracefully like Bill Pearl is doing.

Chart To Use To Calculate Maximal Heart Rate And 80 Percent Of Your Maximal Heart Rate.

Age	Max. Heart Rate	80% Max. Heart Rate
15	205	164
16	204	163
17	203	162
18	202	161
19	201	160
20	200	160
21	199	159
22	198	158
23	197	157
24	196	157
25	195	156
26	194	155
27	193	154
28	192	153
29	191	152
30	190	152
31	189	151
32	188	150
33	187	149
34	186	148
35	185	148

Age	Max. Heart Rate	80% Max. Heart Rate
36	184	147
37	183	146
38	182	145
39	181	144
40	180	144
41	179	143
42	178	142
43	177	141
44	176	140
45	175	140
46	174	139
47	173	138
48	172	137
49	171	136
50	170	136
51	169	135
52	168	134
53	167	133
54	166	132
55	165	132
56	164	131
57	163	130
58	162	129
59	161	128
60	160	128
61	159	127

Age	Max. Heart Rate	80% Max. Heart Rate
62	158	126
63	157	125
64	156	124
65	155	124
66	154	123
67	153	122
68	152	121
69	151	120
70	150	120
71	149	119
72	148	118
73	147	117
74	146	116
75	145	116

Here is the treadmill protocol to determine your functional age.

Time	Miles Per Hour	Elevation (% Grade)
Minutes 1, 2, 3,	1.7	10
Minutes 4, 5, 6	2.5	12
Minutes 7, 8, 9	3.4	14
Minutes 10, 11, 12	4.2	16
Minutes 13, 14, 15	5.0	18
Minutes 16, 17, 18	5.5	20
Minutes 19, 20, 21	6.0	22

Once you choose to grow old vigorously, an exciting world can open up to you. Recharge your batteries with exercise. Normal batteries wear out as the power slowly fades, while recharged batteries produce power at 100 percent until they expend themselves completely. Keep your batteries charged with a SAFE program of strength, aerobics, flexibility and endurance. You needn't be intimidated by exercise. We've all been cut from a team at one point in our lives or we'd all be playing professional sports. Start slowly, you need to use energy to gain energy. If you start aggressively, you'll be too tired. The older you are, the more you should do. Don't use retirement to sit around. Get out! Play a little bit. Make it fun. As the popular saying goes, *Get A Life!*

Don't let the fact that you are older intimidate you. There is absolutely no medical reason for people to stop being active as they age. It's an idea that is as wrong as any old wive's tale, or adage based on misinformation. In the next chapter you'll discover some facts about aging and physical staying power that will astonish you.

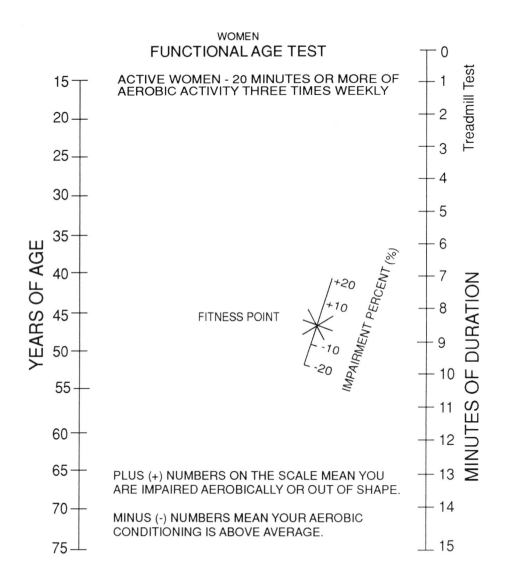

WOMEN
FUNCTIONAL AGE TEST

ACTIVE WOMEN - 20 MINUTES OR MORE OF AEROBIC ACTIVITY THREE TIMES WEEKLY

YEARS OF AGE

15
20
25
30
35
40
45
50
55
60
65
70
75

Treadmill Test

0
1
2
3
4
5
6
7
8
9
10
11
12
13
14
15

MINUTES OF DURATION

FITNESS POINT

+20
+10
-10
-20

IMPAIRMENT PERCENT (%)

PLUS (+) NUMBERS ON THE SCALE MEAN YOU ARE IMPAIRED AEROBICALLY OR OUT OF SHAPE.

MINUS (-) NUMBERS MEAN YOUR AEROBIC CONDITIONING IS ABOVE AVERAGE.

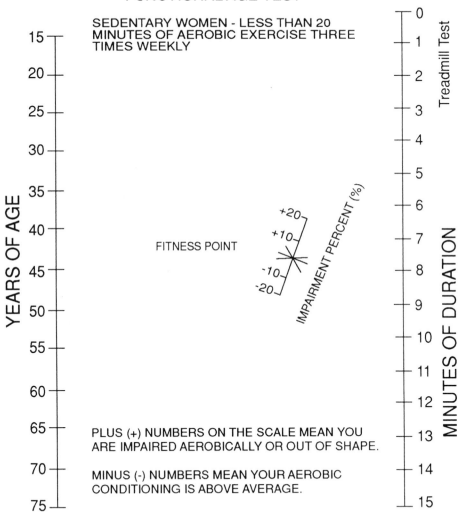

WOMEN
FUNCTIONAL AGE TEST

SEDENTARY WOMEN - LESS THAN 20
MINUTES OF AEROBIC EXERCISE THREE
TIMES WEEKLY

YEARS OF AGE

15
20
25
30
35
40
45
50
55
60
65
70
75

FITNESS POINT

+20
+10
-10
-20

IMPAIRMENT PERCENT (%)

Treadmill Test

MINUTES OF DURATION

0
1
2
3
4
5
6
7
8
9
10
11
12
13
14
15

PLUS (+) NUMBERS ON THE SCALE MEAN YOU
ARE IMPAIRED AEROBICALLY OR OUT OF SHAPE.

MINUS (-) NUMBERS MEAN YOUR AEROBIC
CONDITIONING IS ABOVE AVERAGE.

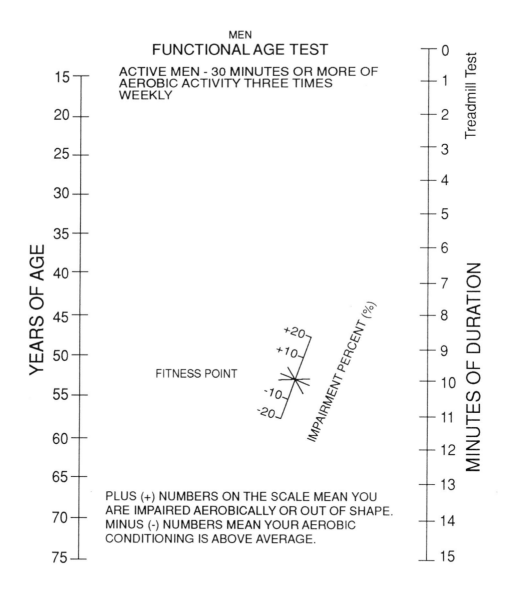

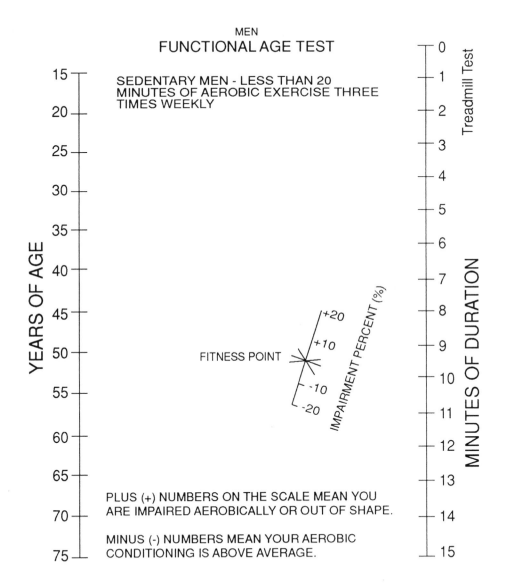

MEN
FUNCTIONAL AGE TEST

SEDENTARY MEN - LESS THAN 20 MINUTES OF AEROBIC EXERCISE THREE TIMES WEEKLY

YEARS OF AGE

15
20
25
30
35
40
45
50
55
60
65
70
75

Treadmill Test

MINUTES OF DURATION

0
1
2
3
4
5
6
7
8
9
10
11
12
13
14
15

+20
+10
-10
-20

FITNESS POINT

IMPAIRMENT PERCENT (%)

PLUS (+) NUMBERS ON THE SCALE MEAN YOU ARE IMPAIRED AEROBICALLY OR OUT OF SHAPE.

MINUS (-) NUMBERS MEAN YOUR AEROBIC CONDITIONING IS ABOVE AVERAGE.

< 14 >

Antigravity Exercises for the Elderly

*Muscle strength can be tripled
in people thought to be too old to stay active.*

Remember years ago when relatives and friends asked you to flex your muscle and you tightened up your biceps? Do it again, now. Bend that elbow while you tighten up the muscle. Now feel that muscle with your other hand. Is it rock hard and firm? Is the skin tight over your biceps or does it hang down below your arm? Is the muscle soft and flabby? Can you pinch the muscle with your opposite thumb and index finger and make a dent?

This easy to find, easy to feel muscle will give you a quick guide to your body's general physical condition. If your biceps is hard with tight skin, chances are that you participate in a regular program of exercise. If your skin hangs down below your arm like your parent's did when they were older, then you need work. Chances are, however, that you are a victim of the myth that aging removes the ability of a person to be strong and agile. *Getting old means losing power.*

Nonsense! Absolute bunk! Certainly, your body slows down, but that does not mean you should give in, and give up. Here are a few facts about aging and strength renewal in the elderly:

Information provided in the June 1992 issue of Nutrition Action News Letter published by Center for Science in the Public Interest quoting research from Tufts University, makes clear that the single most important step to reversal of the aging process is strength training.

By preserving and increasing your muscle mass you can prevent the appearance of the classic signs of aging which are an accumulation of a lifetime of inactivity. The solution is strength training. People aged 65 and older can be made stronger than they've ever been in their lives. A 90-year-old can be made stronger than a 50-year-old. Muscle strength can be tripled in older people.

Thigh muscles are a prime target of improvement in older people because the object is to prevent falls. On a long term basis the goal is to strengthen legs, back muscles, and upper body-arm and chest muscles. The Framingham Heart Study showed that half of women aged 65 can't lift ten pounds. Women have less muscle mass to begin with, and they start to lose muscle strength more rapidly after 60. They can become so profoundly weak that they have to be institutionalized. They become victims of the idea that fragility is a natural outcome of growing old. *It isn't.* Fragility occurs because muscles are neglected.

Gyms that work with older people on strength training start them out at about 60 to 80 percent of their maximum lifting capacity. For nursing home patients, that's about five to ten pounds. In a healthy 65-year-old doing knee exercises, it's about 20 pounds.

Strength training may promote weight-loss as well. The number of calories burned at rest is determined by muscle mass. So the more muscle mass you build, the more calories you burn.

As you saw in Chapter 14, aerobic exercises are also an important part of good health for older people. But researchers at Tufts University said that if they had to choose only one type of exercise to recommend for older people it would be strength training. That's because it has more to do with everyday functional activities. Muscle weakness goes up rapidly after age 70. At age 20, 90 percent of the volume of the thigh is muscle. At age 90, it's only 30 percent muscle. That's one reason the biggest risk to older women is from falling down. With strength training you can increase muscle mass 10 percent, but the increase in strength is 200 percent.

A strength training program is designed to prolong vitality by retarding or even reversing the usual biological deterioration process that people past 45 often begin to experience. Such things as slow down of metabolism, glucose intolerance, and declining strength can be reversed in many cases as the benefits of strength training act to postpone disability by reducing the risk of such chronic conditions as heart disease, Type II diabetes, arteriovascular disease, hypertension,and osteoporosis.

Long-term studies bear out the fact that the average person's lean-body mass declines with age. These studies show that Americans tend to lose about 6.6 pounds of lean-body mass each decade of life. The rate of loss accelerates after age 45. Two things are responsible for how much muscle we have. The first involves how much we use our muscles. The second is the level of tissue-maintaining anabolic hormones circulating in our blood.

How much a muscle is used is partially responsible for its size and lifting capability. Used frequently, a muscle will maintain the status quo. A muscle that is not only used frequently but is pushed to the limits of its capacity will grow and gain strength, even in elderly people. The second muscle-size factor is the amount of anabolic hormones in the bloodstream. Anabolic hormones increase the synthesis of protein. The most potent of these is testosterone. Because men have much more testosterone in their bodies than women, they also have more muscle. Studies have shown that vigorous exercise can cause a phenomenon called "muscle hypertrophy" meaning individual muscle cells grow larger. The same studies offer pretty conclusive evidence that muscle mass and strength can be regained, no matter what your age and no matter what the state of your body's musculature before you start your exercise program.

An eight-week study of 87 to 96 year-old women showed that resistance exercise tripled their muscle strength and increased muscle size by 10 percent. Experience with the old-old-group, (the frail elderly) showed an increase of strength by as much as 190 percent and muscle mass by up to 12 percent by following a program of resistance exercise. This population's quality of life and ability to walk soared.

Older people may be slower to respond to exhortations about exercise, but when they finally do it they are more committed than the typical young adults. Older people tend to circle around the idea of exercise for a while before they commit themselves. Just remember that the primary goal of weight training is to keep people independent through exercise. There is no substitute. Does strength training mean that you should neglect regular exercise? Of course not. Exercise is the central ingredient of good health. To be really effective, it should be combined with strength and flexibility training. Exercise tones the muscles, strengthens the bones, makes the heart and lungs work better, and helps prevent constipation. It increases physical reserve and vitality. The increased reserve function helps you deal with crises. Exercise eases depression, aids sleep, and enhances activities of daily life.

Here are simple family-room strength improvement exercises to tone your major muscles and fight the effects of gravity that seem to be pulling every part of your body down toward the earth. Instead of 44-inch chests becoming 44-inch abdomens, let's start your antigravity program. All you need is a rope and a chair. Use these exercises when you are waiting in the car for a few minutes. Leave a rope in the car for those times you are waiting for someone else and want to use the time efficiently.

Arms—Biceps and Triceps.

Sit in your favorite chair and wrap the rope around your back like you see in illustration 135. Isometrically or without movement, pull the rope forward while you feel the muscles on the back of your arms tighten. Hold this position for eight seconds, then relax. This strengthens the Triceps or back of the upper arm muscles. Do three to five sets.

The Biceps.

Sit in your chair and put the rope under your feet as you see in illustration 136. Grasp the ends of the rope and pull upward. The rope won't move but your muscles will be working and you will feel them tightening. Do this for eight seconds.

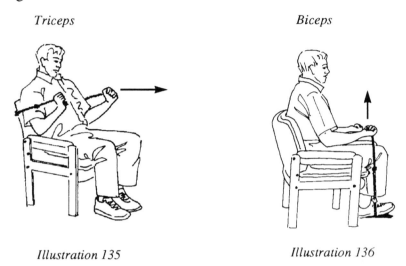

Triceps   *Biceps*

Illustration 135   *Illustration 136*

Back Muscles.

Sit on a couch or soft chair, not in a recliner. With your feet flat on the floor, push backward into the back of the chair with your back. You'll feel the muscles contract as you start to push into the cushions. The muscles will tighten and strengthen. Hold for eight seconds then relax. Illustration 140A.

Abdominal Muscles.

This test is similar to the triceps test except you wrap the rope around the chair then twist it a few times snug against your chest. Now push forward with your upper body against the rope for eight seconds. Since the rope is twisted a few times, it won't slip. Hold for eight seconds. Illustration 138.

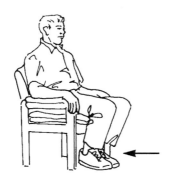

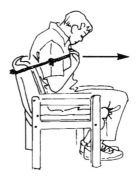

Illustration 137

Hamstring

Illustration 138

Abdominal

Thigh Muscles. Illustration 139.

The quadriceps or front thigh muscle can be toughened up by crossing your feet in front of your favorite chair. Plant your left foot in the carpet. Now put your right foot behind your left foot and push forward with your right foot while pulling back with your planted left foot. Repeat with the opposite leg.

Hamstring or Back of Thigh Muscles.

While in your favorite chair, pull your legs back against the chair. Pull with both legs for eight seconds. Feel the muscles tighten on the back of the thigh and knee. Illustration 137.

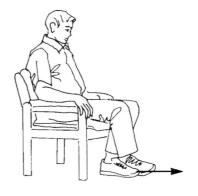

Illustration 139

Thigh

Rotary Torso—Twister.

With your back pressed gently into the back of your chair, twist slowly to the right while pushing your right shoulder into the chair; at the same time tighten your abdominal muscles. Hold for eight seconds. Repeat on the opposite side. This will firm up the side abdominal muscles.

Illustration 140

A   B

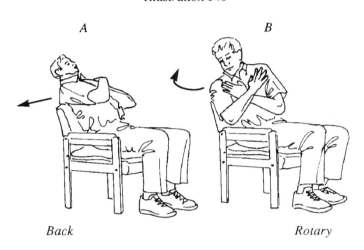

Back   Rotary

In less than one minute you've started on the road to recovery—one day at a time. Repeat these exercises during TV commercials or when you finish a magazine article or after reading a chapter in a book. A few weeks from now you'll feel the changes taking place. You'll have more bounce for the stairs, you'll feel firmer and you'll be starting to take control of your life.

You may discover that you will be interested in developing a more sophisticated strength training program. If that is the case, be certain to talk with an experienced strength trainer at the gym of your choice before you commence a serious, advanced program.

< 15 >

Questions I Am Frequently Asked By Back Pain Patients

Don't be surprised at some of the answers;
they prove the back can be trained to recover from injury.

1.   *How long should I ride in the car?*

Sitting increases the pressure on the discs of the back. Since the back is made to move and sitting does not encourage maximum blood flow, I recommend that for every hour stop for at least five minutes. Flex, bend backwards, and twist. Walk around for a few minutes to increase blood flow.

2.   *Will a water bed help?*

Newer water beds have baffles or separations in the mattress that allow for good back support if the mattress has enough water in it. For long-term back problems, the heat of the water bed may help decrease your morning stiffness.

3.   *A back brace makes my back feel better, but when I take it off my back hurts more. What should I do?*
Weight lifters and workers in heavy lifting industries like home movers wear back support belts when moving heavy objects. These leather or woven belts do provide back protection when lifting but if they are worn all the time, they do some of the stabilizing work that the spine muscles should be doing. The result: your back muscles become weaker when you are trying to make them strong. The belts are only for temporary help, they are not for constant wear.

4.   *When is back pain serious?*
Back pain can be worrisome, but is serious when you have problems with bladder or bowel control, when your foot scrapes with walking, feels weak or when the pain is excruciating. If any of these symptoms occur, then see your doctor immediately.

5.   *How can I stop the pain?*
When you are experiencing a flare-up of symptoms, then put into action the acronym AIMS, which stands for aspirin or anti-inflammatory, ice, massage and stretching. Chapter 8 has specific information on this protocol.

6.   *If I have surgery, how will my back function without the disc?*
The spine can function very well without the disc since the tough circular fibers around the disc can act as cushions for your everyday activities.

7.   *Why should I want to exercise when my back hurts?*
When your back is sore, it seems ridiculous to exercise, but exercise is frequently the one activity that will help decrease back pain later. If the back

is not used, it stiffens up. It can't be in spasm and be stretched at the same time, so as you stretch it the spasm will decrease and the tightness will decrease.

8.   *My doctor said to rest in bed for two weeks when my back hurts—it seems to help. Why should I exercise?*

Two or three days of bed rest may help with inflammation and strained muscles but additional rest will only cause the muscles to soften. Your pain will decrease but with the loss of three percent of your back strength for each day of rest past three days, you will be more likely to be injured in the future. Exercise will prevent loss of back strength.

9.   *Anti-inflammatory medications irritate my stomach so I can't take them. What can I do?*

Non-prescription ibuprofen is only one kind of anti-inflammatory. Several others are available from your doctor. If you have a sensitive stomach, ask you doctor about CYTOTEC, a newer agent that protects the stomach from anti-inflammatory medications.

10.   *If I start a therapy program, how long will it take to "fix" my back?*

Functional restoration programs take one to three months depending on the severity of your symptoms. If your doctor recommends an active therapy program, then go. It may change your life.

11.   *Can I have a new disc put in my back?*

The new replacement discs show promise, but for now they are still experimental and have shown a lot of problems, including release of metal shavings into the area around the spine. Focus on what you can do without trying experimental surgery.

12.   *What should I expect when I see a spine doctor?*

For your first visit expect to spend one to two hours for a detailed history of your problem followed by a physical examination with special focus on the back. X-rays will be reviewed or additional ones may be taken. You may receive computerized spine strength testing. A diagnosis will be made and you will be given directions about treatment options such as physical therapy and exercise, biofeedback to learn how to relax your muscles, and injection techniques to help calm an inflamed nerve. Low current electrical stimulation from small AA batteries may help break the pain cycle or you may be sent for additional tests such as magnetic resonance scans to better evaluate your back.

It takes time if you have a complicated problem, so give your doctor the time he or she needs to pinpoint the problem.

13.   *Who should I see if I have back pain? What do all the initials mean behind the names?*

It may seem confusing that you have multiple choices for treatment, but here they are:

An M.D. is the typical doctor you think of when someone mentions going to a physician or doctor.

A D.O. is a Doctor of Osteopathic medicine, a physician qualified and licensed to perform the same services as an M.D. and who has more focus relative to the musculoskeletal system during his medical training.

D.C. stands for Doctor of Chiropractic. The Doctor of Chiropractic spends all of his training working with problems of the musculoskeletal system. He performs manipulation and physiotherapy.

N.D. means Doctor of Naturopathy. Naturopathy deals with therapy by natural means such as fresh air and exercise, physiotherapy, manipulation and the use of herbs in place of medications.

P.T. refers to Physical Therapist. In most states, the Physical Therapist carries out orders of a physician. The typical therapy he or she performs has been mentioned. The P.T. is the major player in functional restoration.

M.T. stands for Massage Therapist. It is a branch of natural health care that involves manipulation of muscles and other soft tissues of the body, relaxation and the teaching of self-care.

To complicate everything, there are subdivisions in each of the areas of medical care. Sports medicine encompasses all of these areas at times and you may find any combination of the above working together. Often a D.C. or N.D. will employ a Massage Therapist, or an M.D. or D.O. will work with a Physical Therapist, or Massage Therapist.

In addition, your caregiver may focus on restoration or may have special training in surgery of back problems.

Ask the following questions of your caregiver.

1. What is your main focus of therapy?
2. Do you do functional restoration?
3. What is my role in recovering the use of my back?
4. What special training do you have to help my back problem?
5. How much time will you spend with me while I am involved in rehab?
6. Can you release me to work part-time while I am in rehab?
7. Does insurance pay for your services?
8. What should I expect during therapy?
9. Is there a back school to learn more about my back?
10. Are the tests measurable and reproducible?
11. Can I return to my regular job at completion of the therapy?
12. How can I measure my progress along the way?
13. What if I develop more pain during the program?

These questions will give you a beginning in your discussions regarding your recovery.

In spite of the differences in training, your primary concern is who can help you. A physician involved with rehab may be your best choice. There are many specialty areas for M.D.'s, D.O.'s, N.D.'s and D.C.'s, These specialty areas may be restoration, sports medicine, radiology, research, or any number of other possibilities. You still need to answer the thirteen questions above. Talk to your insurance claims examiner for suggestions. If you know someone who was hurt and who went through a low back rehabilitation program and who now is working and functioning normally, talk to her or him. Also listen to the advice of your physician or therapist.

14. What kind of schedule should I adopt following an injury?

The first four weeks after an injury follow the advice of your doctor and use the first aid ideas mentioned earlier. The suggestion was to use the memory aid "AIMS". A is for aspirin, I is for ice, M is for massage and S is for stretching. Of all four of these, stretching is the most important. Go to physical therapy if it is recommended. Ask your employer if you can work part-time or light-duty for a while if it is okay with your physician. Do all the prescribed exercises and stretches recommended. Ask your doctor or therapist if more time spent on these home exercises and stretching will be of more benefit and if so, do them.

During this therapy period, it may seem that your doctor is not doing much. Follow all the suggestions. Don't skip your appointments even though it seems your doctor is not doing much. He or she is monitoring your therapy and will make any needed changes.

If after six weeks you still are having problems, sit down with your doctor and make a plan for the next six weeks. Included in this should be consideration of a functional restoration program. Some but not all doctors know about these programs.

What does a functional restoration program do? Obviously, it helps you to restore function to your back. How does it do this?

The early steps will be a physical examination followed by computerized testing of your back and abdominal muscles. These machines are designed to test specific muscle groups in the low back and abdomen and to show how much deterioration of muscle strength and flexibility has occurred. These tests are reproducible and reliable.

Following this, a program will be developed for you requiring two or three hours of effort per day three times per week in a structured program. There will be basic exercises and stretches and then specific strengthening exercises and stretches for you plus you will get instruction in a back school.

This program will last from four to twelve weeks depending on how quickly you return to normal function. During the process, you will be doing strengthening exercises for your back and abdominal muscles that contribute to the integrity of your low back.

You will have the testing repeated and will be able to see your increased strength and function on computer-generated printouts. Examples of machines that may be used to measure strength throughout the range of motion of your back and abdomen include:

     1. Medx Computerized Machines.
     2. Nautilus Computerized Machines.
     3. Cybex Computerized Machines.
     4. Kin-Com System.
     5. Lido System.
     6. Biodex Back Attachment.
     7. Others are in development.

It will be exciting to finally see measurable improvement in your back. During this period, you will be encouraged to work part-time or do light-duty work.

In the pyramid of low back pain, I mentioned that most back pain goes away in six months but that there is a 70 percent chance of having another injury within one year. If you graduate from a functional rehab program, you will not be any more likely to injure your back again than a person without any previous injury. The program will help you get off the pain pyramid altogether.

In the rehab program, you will find it refreshing that you are put in a position of responsibility for your back. The recovery is up to you. The therapists are with you continually urging you on and helping you to do the program correctly and the physician is monitoring your activities carefully. You have a supportive crew to work with but the brunt of the work is up to you. Your program will be specific so you will always know what to do. Never hesitate to ask questions about your back, about the machines, or about the program.

One aspect of the program that is helpful is the back school for education. The back school will review the anatomy, the function of an injured back, and how to best benefit from the program. The program aims at modifying pain behavior and teaching self-responsibility for your back. Also included are instructions to show you the proper techniques for lifting and performing the activities of daily life.

You will be taught the proper methods for determining your appropriate heart rate during exercise. A heart rate that is too slow will not allow proper training of the heart and lungs. A heart rate that is too rapid will result in over-training with fatigue and muscle pain.

Nutrition basics will be stressed to help you make better choices on eating to help you lose some of the weight that you probably gained after your injury. After all, we continue to eat the same even if we decrease our activity and this causes the weight gain. We suggest you pick up a 25 pound weight. This is the average extra weight most of us carry around with us. Try carrying the weight around with you for thirty minutes. Losing this 25 pounds can make a tremendous difference in how you feel.

You'll need to review the stretches and how to do them. If they are not done correctly, you will lose much of the benefit of the program. As you approach the end of the program, you will be given time to discuss what happens next. You will be referred to a fitness center in your area with a specific program to maintain fitness and strength. Remember the SAFE approach to rehab: Strength, Aerobics, Flexibility, and Education. If there is no local fitness facility, you will be given guidance to purchase the appropriate home equipment and you will be shown how to use it to your best advantage.

This book contains many home exercises and pool therapy if you have access to a pool. Pool therapy is usually used early in treatment of an injury, but it is also a gentle stretching program that puts minimal strain on your back.

You will be followed and retested by the functional restoration facility to make sure that you are maintaining appropriate strength and flexibility.

15. *What can you expect now that you have completed the program?*

Since you have finished this program, you will have a much better understanding about your back. You will feel assured that you are not likely to reinjure your back. You will know that once in a while you will have a flare-up of back pain and you will know how to deal quickly with the flare-up. *You will be in control.*

Your pain will be much improved. You may still have some pain but you will have learned how to deal with it. You will be enthusiastic about your new body and the feelings which have developed. You'll feel self-assured and will walk with a firm step. You'll stop worrying about your back. You know that your back won't let you down.

These self-assured feelings will give you a new outlook on your life, and your work. Functional restoration rehabs your life and not just your back.

Back injuries add $1,800.00 to the cost of each car produced in the U.S. The money is minor compared to the chronic pain, loss of jobs and inability to enjoy sports and recreation. The quality of life is often impaired tremendously.

The goal of functional restoration is to work-harden your body as you recover from your back injury. The S.A.F.E. program works to cure the problem, not the symptoms. The rapid increase in Strength, Aerobics, Flexibility along with the Education will spark a feeling of hope that helps you grow into a highly-motivated person. The wellness lifestyle stresses weight loss, stress management, and goal setting.

You will be able to accomplish more in less time and will be able to function again in your family, your job, and in your community. You will "ARMOR-PLATE" your back against future problems.

About The Author

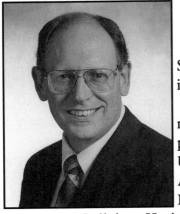

Timothy J. Gray, D.O. is the medical director of Spinecare Of The Pacific and is in private practice in Forest Grove, Oregon.

Previously, he was medical director of a spine rehabilitation clinic in Beaverton, Oregon. He is past instructor of Human Anatomy at Pacific University and at present is a member of the American Osteopathic College of Rehabilitation Medicine and the American Osteopathic Academy of Sports Medicine. He is a clinical assistant professor for the College of Osteopathic Medicine of the Pacific. Dr. Gray has worked with Western Medical Consultants as an independent medical evaluator for spine conditions and has been a medical disability consultant for the Oregon State Insurance Commission. Dr. Gray has published several health-related articles.

He is a member of the American Osteopathic Association, the Osteopathic Physicians and Surgeons of Oregon, the Oregon Medical Association, and the American Medical Association. He graduated with a B.S. degree from the University of Dayton, and took his medical training at Kirksville College of Osteopathic Medicine where he was admitted to Sigma Phi, the honorary society for the advancement of osteopathic medicine. He took his internship and internal medicine training at Doctors Hospital in Columbus, Ohio.

Doctor Gray has treated more than 5,000 back-injured patients including employees of INTEL, Safeway and Albertsons as well as members of the Professional Golf Association.

To order additional copies of
Back Works

Please send ____ copies at $15.95 each book, plus $2 shipping and handling for the first book, $1 for each additional book in the same order.

Enclosed is my check or money order of $_____

or   [ ] Visa [ ] MasterCard

#_____ Exp. Date _____

Signature _____

Name _____

Street Address_____

City _____

State _____ Zip _____

(Advise if recipient and mailing address is different from above.)

Return this order form to:

BookPartners, Inc.
P.O. Box 19732
Seattle, Washington 98109
1-800-925-9881

PROGRESS CHART OF BACK TEST RESULTS

	Date	Points
Spine Strength Testing	_____	_____
Flexibility Testing		
Back flexion	_____	_____
Back extension	_____	_____
Side bending right	_____	_____
Side bending left	_____	_____
Rotation right	_____	_____
Rotation left	_____	_____
Straight leg raise right	_____	_____
Straight leg raise left	_____	_____
Knee to chest right	_____	_____
Knee to chest left	_____	_____
Total Flexibility Points	_____	_____
Endurance Testing		
Upper abdomen	_____	_____
Lower abdomen	_____	_____
Upper lumbar	_____	_____
Lower lumbar	_____	_____
Quadriceps	_____	_____
Total Endurance Points	_____	_____
Total Aerobic Points	_____	_____

Total Spine Strength   _____ +
Aerobic Points   _____ +
Flexibility   _____ +
Endurance   _____ =
_____ Divide by 4 for Score _____

PROGRESS CHART OF BACK TEST RESULTS

	Date	Points
Spine Strength Testing	_____	_____
Flexibility Testing		
Back flexion	_____	_____
Back extension	_____	_____
Side bending right	_____	_____
Side bending left	_____	_____
Rotation right	_____	_____
Rotation left	_____	_____
Straight leg raise right	_____	_____
Straight leg raise left	_____	_____
Knee to chest right	_____	_____
Knee to chest left	_____	_____
Total Flexibility Points	_____	_____
Endurance Testing		
Upper abdomen	_____	_____
Lower abdomen	_____	_____
Upper lumbar	_____	_____
Lower lumbar	_____	_____
Quadriceps	_____	_____
Total Endurance Points	_____	_____
Total Aerobic Points	_____	_____

Total Spine Strength   _____ +
Aerobic Points   _____ +
Flexibility   _____ +
Endurance   _____ =
_____ Divide by 4 for Score _____